A NEW AMERICAN
ACUPUNCTURE

A NEW AMERICAN ACUPUNCTURE

ACUPUNCTURE OSTEOPATHY

The Myofascial Release
of the Bodymind's
Holding Patterns

by

Mark Seem

BLUE POPPY PRESS

Published by:
BLUE POPPY PRESS
A Division of Blue Poppy Enterprises, Inc.
5441 Western Ave., Suite 2
BOULDER, CO 80301

First Edition, May, 1993
Second Printing, October, 1993
Third Printing, June, 1994
Fourth Printing, October, 1995
Fifth Printing, May, 1996
Sixth Printing, May, 1997
Seventh Printing, November, 1999
Eighth Printing, September, 2003
Ninth Printing, July, 2004
Tenth Printing, October, 2005
Eleventh Printing, September, 2006
Twelvth Printing, March, 2007
Thirteenth Printing, February, 2008
Fourteenth Printing, March, 2009

ISBN 0-936185-44-9
ISBN 978-0-936185-44-6
LC 93-71097

DISCLAIMER: The information in this book is given in good faith. However, the author and the publishers cannot be held responsible for any error or omission. The publishers will not accept liabilities for any injuries or damages caused to the reader that may result from the reader's acting upon or using the content contained in this book. The publishers make this information available to English language readers for research and scholarly purposes only.

The publishers do not advocate nor endorse self-medication by laypersons. Chinese medicine is a professional medicine. Laypersons interested in availing themselves of the treatments described in this book should seek out a qualified professional practitioner of Chinese medicine.

COMP Designation: Original work

20 19 18 17 16 15 14 13

Cover design by Anne Rue

Printed at Hess Print Solutions, Woodstock, Illinois

Preface

Acupuncture pain management should be a routine part of any acupuncture student's training, and the public at large should be right in assuming, as they do, that acupuncturists are highly effective in the treatment of pain and its various dysfunctions. The American Medical Association itself has listed acupuncture as an appropriate adjunctive therapy for pain management, and the treatment of recurrent and chronic pain has been discussed in the medical literature as one of our most pressing and costly health care concerns.

Yet many acupuncturists freely admit that, while they can treat acute pain effectively and rapidly, chronic pain more often than not fails to improve in any significant fashion using the currently dominant acupuncture methodology. When teaching at various schools and conferences from the West Coast to England, one of the most frequent questions I am asked revolves around the treatment of chronic pain, and I am often struck by the lack of training in this area at most Western acupuncture schools.

This even began to happen at the school I founded and still direct, the Tri-State Institute of Traditional Chinese Acupuncture. Several years ago, I stepped back from regular clinical supervision of my students. At that time, I was preoccupied with my work for the National Council of Acupuncture Schools and Colleges (NCASC) and the National Commission for the Certification of Acupuncturists (NCCA). The chief clinical supervisor to whom I turned over my clinical duties had recently returned from extensive post-graduate training in the People's Republic of China (PRC). Therefore, I naively felt I was leaving our third-year clinical interns in good hands. Nonetheless, I scheduled myself to do clinical supervision every three months so that I could still check on our student interns' development.

At my first such clinical supervision, I began to feel very uneasy. A number of interns asked to see me in the conference area to discuss the patients they were treating. Typically, they gave me a detailed explanation of what the patient was suffering from and their acupuncture diagnosis and treatment plan which they wanted me to approve. On the one hand, it all sounded very professional. On the other, I was disturbed by what I was hearing. A few hours into the day, I started telling students that, until I saw the patients for myself, I had no idea if their diagnoses and treatment plans were appropriate.

I then started going from treatment cubicle to treatment cubicle evaluating their patients. That is when I realized our students had no idea of how to touch the bodies of their patients to directly assess the status of these patients' meridian systems. Whereas I diagnose and treat based primarily on palpation of strategic acupuncture points and meridians to determine where qi is stagnant, these students were only palpating the radial artery pulse, looking at the tongue, and asking questions without otherwise touching their patients' bodies. I was appalled, and it took me quite a while to realize that the fault lay in the tcm, internal, herbal medicine perspective our supervisor had brought back, wholesale and uncritically, from the PRC.

At first I became angry over the pervasive influence TCM has had on American acupuncture. Over the last eight years or so, this style of acupuncture has insinuated itself into every American acupuncture school curriculum and served as the focus of the NCCA examination. I believe this style ignores the complexity of the acupuncture meridian system which is the basis of the French acupuncture I had originally learned and was, in turn, attempting to teach to my students. In my experience, once one has had too great a taste of TCM acupuncture with its heady logic, facile abstractions, and even more facile repetitive point combinations, a hands-on, meridian-based approach often seems inferior.

As I continued to clarify my ideas about and experience of acupuncture, it became clear to me that a hands-on approach emphasizing palpation of constricted areas of the body is fundamental in the practice of meridian acupuncture. That is when I urged my faculty, a few of whom disagreed strongly, to bring in Kiiko Matsumoto. Kiiko Matsumoto is one of the main teachers of Japanese meridian acupuncture in the United States. She had been teaching occasional weekend workshops for us, but now I wanted to make her a regular clinical supervisor. The faculty critical of this plan felt it would confuse students by introducing them to yet another system. This group felt that TCM should be the focus of our curriculum. I argued, however, that Kiiko's Japanese meridian acupuncture would instill a clinical pragmatism in our training which was lacking in TCM acupuncture. It would also show our students that there are many different options for treating from a meridian acupuncture perspective, and that palpation is central in such an approach.

After several years, I rejoined the clinical faculty on a regular basis and, after we brought in other senior supervisors trained in yet other acupuncture styles, I became less angry at TCM acupuncture. Within this more dispassionate space, I have been able to continue to refine my analysis of and differentiation between TCM and meridian-based acupuncture. I have continued to study and practice French, Vietnamese, and Japanese meridian-based acupuncture systems and have integrated these with Western research and practice concerning trigger points. Thus I have developed my own style of acupuncture which emphasizes the immediate release of areas of palpable constriction using a combination of distal points selected on the basis of meridian theory and local points selected by touch.

During the last several years, my mission for both myself and my school has become clear. I want to show how powerful acupuncture is as a therapy and especially for recurrent and chronic pain conditions *when it is practiced from its own, meridian-based perspective*. Where TCM acupuncture takes the palpable, felt body out of acupuncture, a meridian-based system of acupuncture puts it back in. In our modern medical climate where touch has been removed from medicine and been replaced by sterile objective tests, I feel meridian acupuncture can insert itself and, thereby, re-establish informed touch as both a powerful diagnostic tool and a safe and effective therapeutic methodology.

This book on the treatment of recurrent and chronic pain from a meridian-based acupuncture perspective has arisen out of the many questions students and graduates have asked when I have demonstrated my treatment of pain. While such questions should be unnecessary for well-trained acupuncturists, it is my experience that the ability to successfully treat chronic pain has been lost for those not trained in a meridian-based approach. The famous physician Sun Si-miao stressed the need to treat *a shi* (tender) points when treating pain conditions because these points, not the textbook ones, are where the qi has become blocked and stagnant. What is acupuncture if not treatment to regulate the flow of qi through the meridian systems of the organism by releasing blockages on the surface of the body?

When I learned a few years ago of the seminal work on trigger, *i.e.,* tender, points by Dr. Janet Travell and began studying it, I realized she had rediscovered, from a Western myofascial rather than an Oriental meridian perspective, exactly what Sun Si-miao meant. In the following text, I hope to convey the spirit of this rediscovery of tender points and the crucial role acupuncture can play in mainstream pain management.

MDS
Fire Island, NY
August 1992

Contents

Part II: Treatment Protocols

Introduction

The Point of Acupuncture

In Traditional Chinese Medicine or TCM's attempt to standardize Chinese medicine into a unified system that could be taught in identical fashion to countless numbers of students throughout the People's Republic of China's new Institutes of Traditional Chinese Medicine starting in the early 1960s, the mainland Chinese also standardized the locations of the acupuncture points in Western scientific, anatomical terms. Rather than the vague classical definitions, such as, "in a depression a hand's breadth below the outside of the knee", Chinese TCM acupuncturists with an eye to the West sought something far more rigorous. In carrying out this standardization, acupuncture points were laid over the various anatomical images of muscles, nerves, blood vessels, and bones from their Western atlases. The charts which made their way to the West showed beautifully rendered images of the nervous system, the circulatory system, the muscular system, and the skeletal system with the acupuncture points drawn in precisely. At the same time, TCM acupuncture textbooks translated from Chinese leaned and still lean heavily toward the skeletal image with their precise descriptions of bones, tendons, and joints. Most TCM textbook locations thus recharted the vaguely defined classical point locations onto this seemingly more precise and scientifically sound backdrop.

In looking at classical Chinese diagrams of point location, however, one sees no such attempts at anatomical precision. No muscles are drawn in, not even shadings to indicate key muscular configurations and bony protuberances. All that appears in these totally flat drawings is a general pathway of a specific meridian with a specific number of points drawn in for each. It would seem that these early charts were meant, along with the vague descriptions of point location that accompanied them in the early texts, as a mere guide to enable the student to learn the basic pathways, the number of points, and the general point locations for each meridian. Then the student was expected to find a teacher who would demonstrate how to palpate the surface of the body, feeling along meridian pathways until something was felt under the fingertips that indicated that the actual point lay precisely there. This early, oral tradition required a close teacher-student relationship and assumed that much that is essential to the successful practice of acupuncture had to be felt directly and not just memorized from diagrams and books.

This method of experience-based point location changed dramatically once the standard Western anatomical locations were established in contemporary TCM textbooks. Point locations in such books are now given as, "at the midpoint of the transverse crease of the popliteal fossa, between the tendons of m. biceps femoris and m. semitendinosus," or, "1.5 *cun* lateral to the lower border of the spinous process of the 3rd thoracic vertebra."[1] While these descriptions appear very precise, they do not state what muscle the acupuncture needle actually penetrates or is imbedded in. For instance, in the first case above, the needle is imbedded in the plantaris muscle, the actual site of Bl 40; while in the second case, the needle is embedded in the superficial paraspinal, erector spinae muscles, the actual muscular site of the back *shu* points like Bl 13 above. Opting primarily for a skeletal image of point location, contemporary TCM leads its students of acupuncture away from a knowledge of the body that has to be touched to be known toward one that can simply be measured. In a now seemingly scientific fashion, acupuncture students have become skilled at rapid location of points measured against exact textbook locations.

---

1   *Essentials of Chinese Acupuncture,* Foreign Languages Press, Beijing, 1980, p. 187 and 178 respectively

There is a major problem here, of course. The needle is not inserted into the "midpoint of the transverse crease of the popliteal fossa" between two tendons *but into the plantaris muscle.* Nor is a needle inserted into a place "1.5 *cun* lateral to the lower border of the spinous process of the 3rd thoracic vertebra" *but into the superficial paraspinal, erector spinae muscles at that level.* Acupuncture needles are inserted into muscular and connective soft tissue, not simply into spaces between bones and tendons. When a needle succeeds in creating the celebrated *de qi* response indicating the "arrival of qi," the needle has actually caused a myofascial response whereby the muscle underlying the needle begins to contract and "grasp" the needle.

If TCM picked the wrong anatomical image for the location of acupuncture points when it settled on the skeletal one, perhaps this is because the task itself, establishing precise anatomical point locations, was ill-conceived in the first place. If it had selected a myofascial anatomical image instead and then focused on what the practitioner was going to feel once the needle was inserted, *i.e.*, needle grasp, it would have been obliged to provide a different sort of point location. This sort of location would have to indicate what muscle the point was located in and what the tissue should feel like there. This is, I believe, how point location is taught in Japan where what is felt guides what is needled.

But is this really such a big deal? I think so. Let me back up to the days when I was first learning how to needle acupuncture points on patients. Concerned about safety and wishing to become as grounded as possible in point location and needling, for which my education in French philosophy had certainly never prepared me, I asked another student, a medical doctor, to assist me. I asked her to hold the body where I was going to needle and to tell me what was really going on when the inserted needle produced the characteristic dull, distending, achy sensation. I needled LI 4 and felt something very specific. I asked my physician peer what really happened, and she said the muscle just jumped a bit and was now grabbing the needle.

And so I retained, from that moment on, a muscular image of what I was doing when I inserted needles into the bodies of my patients.

Our teachers at Lincoln Acupuncture Detox, who had trained at the Quebec Institute of Acupuncture with Oscar and Mario Wexu in a very hands-on, physical style of acupuncture, made students do what they had done in Montreal. This consisted of massaging every patient for several minutes before administering acupuncture in order to free up tight muscular constrictions and ready the body for the needles. I, therefore, learned from the start to find tight spots in the muscles, and these are what we needled most frequently. When they were needled, the muscles would quiver, twitch, or even jump quite dramatically. I could feel this with my left hand, which we were taught to keep on the patient with the index and middle fingers straddling the located point. This *left-handed knowledge*, I came to realize, is a big part of acupuncture education and is easily taught if a myofascial image is the focus.

Little did I know at that time that most acupuncturists do not share this myofascial, meridian-based image of point location and needling. I was quite good at point location and needling straight away. Therefore, none of my teachers or colleagues ever questioned what I was doing. While they had been taught a hands-on, myofascial approach, the new TCM texts from the PRC were providing more precise anatomical locations which everyone felt compelled to commit to memory. This situation led rather quickly to a replication of TCM acupuncture point location, and shortly thereafter to point formularies in the United States. Many people trained in non-TCM or pre-TCM styles, as we had been in Quebec, started speaking the TCM language as well, and state and national examinations followed suit.

Perhaps this is why I valued Kiiko Matsumoto's teaching from her very first weekend at my school. She made it clear that she was not practicing TCM acupuncture, and it was clear in watching her that palpation of the body was her focus for diagnosis, point location, and treatment. When Matsumoto and Birch's *Hara Diagnosis*:

Reflections on the Sea[2] appeared, I rejoiced. Here was a highly articulate case made for viewing acupuncture as a myofascial, connective tissue therapy. According to Matsumoto and Birch, when muscles and soft connective tissue are needled, there is not only release of the myofascial body, but the skeletal system also responds. In addition, the major systems of the body—nervous, arterial, circulatory, and lymphatic—all can communicate more freely.

At that time, chiropractors studying at my school would often express amazement that treatment of tight points in the muscles led to such rapid and sustained skeletal release, often even more effectively than chiropractic adjustments. Their responses led me to study the principles of osteopathic and physical medicine in seminars and publications from the Upledger Institute and in the writings of other osteopaths and physical therapists. Thus I grew more and more fascinated with the concepts of myofascial release of the body's holding patterns. I was certain that acupuncture as I understood it was a powerful myofascial therapy in that sense. For instance, A. T. Still, the founder of modern Western osteopathy, defined the osteopathic equivalent of acupuncture imaging as follows: "A normal image of the form and function must be seen by the mind's eye or our work will condemn us."[3]

Meridian-based acupuncture or acupuncture seen from an acupuncture systems point of view is similar in intent to Still's osteopathy. Acupuncture thus conceived effects a physical manipulation of the body the same as in Still's vision and practice. This physical manipulation, achieved by inserting needles into the muscles and connective tissue, frees up the normal flow of blood, energy, and nutrients by releasing myofascial and musculoskeletal constrictions. Still's

---

[2]   Matsumoto, Kiiko and Birch, Stephen, *Hara Diagnosis: Reflections on the Sea*, Paradigm Publications, Brookline, MA, 1988

[3]   Still, A. T., *Osteopathy: Research & Practice,* Eastland Press, Seattle, 1992, p. 21

vision of the practice of osteopathy is equally valid when applied to a meridian-based, myofascial practice of acupuncture: "As an engineer you see friction, as a philosopher you conclude there is an obstruction and as a mechanic you remove the obstruction."[4] Thus, the release of myofascial and musculoskeletal obstruction to restore normal flow through acupuncture needling is, in a sense, *acupuncture osteopathy*.

I have chosen this admittedly dramatic subtitle to make this point: Acupuncture from a meridian perspective is primarily a myofascial, musculoskeletal therapy. Nonetheless, it catalyzes the added indirect benefits of any such myofascial therapy, namely the improvement of internal function and the nourishment of the organism. Western-style medical research, in both Asia and the West, has shown that acupuncture can affect many internal changes. These changes can account biomedically for how acupuncture affects what seem to be internal medical problems. However, my point is that acupuncture does this by treating the body surface or the myofascial body fabric.

When needles are inserted, holding patterns in the body fabric are stimulated. During the first few minutes, these appear to grow even more strained. The tight, dull, vibratory sensations experienced by patients during the first few minutes of acupuncture treatment might well be due to the additional strain the needles have introduced into this holding pattern. Nonetheless, as this strain builds up or increases, it leads to eventual release. This process may also be stated as a type of strain/counterstrain.

I believe acupuncture needles lead the body to respond with its various healing changes because we, as acupuncturists, primarily affect the body's connective tissue. The irritation of needling leads this tissue to respond and, I believe, it is this response that leads to all sorts

---

4   *Ibid.*, p. 25

of other internal and external changes. Even when one wants to make the most profound, internal changes, for example, to calm an unregulated nervous and immune system in chronic fatigue syndrome, in my opinion, an acupuncturist's focus should remain on the surface of the patient's body, on the sites where the needles are inserted.

There are those acupuncturists who will inevitably respond that comparisons of acupuncture to osteopathy or physical therapy downgrade the ancient art of acupuncture. I recommend these critics to read A. T. Still. He expected his osteopathy to be able to treat the vast majority of human conditions, including internal medical conditions. Nevertheless, he stressed over and over the need to be a good engineer able to detect a system working on overdrive, creating friction and excess; a pragmatic philosopher able to trace back from the friction to the site of obstruction; and a good mechanic able to release this obstruction. The method in his system was the physical manipulation of hard and soft tissue. Viewed from this perspective, I believe the mkst important method in acupuncture is the insertion of needles to induce a myofascial response or release.

The next stage in my own development of a myofascial style of meridian-based acupuncture was my encounter with the work of Dr. Janet Travell. Her work on the release of tender trigger points to treat myofascial pain and dysfunction is the foundation of modern physical medicine and rehabilitation's management of pain. Her story is that of a pioneer who refused the wisdom of her day to envision an entirely different picture of what pain was all about. Most people in the first half of this century believed complex or chronic pain disorders with no objective or organic cause were psychosomatic and better referred to psychotherapy. Travell was convinced they were myofascial and required physical therapy. In the process, she rediscovered the whole story of tender points so eloquently elaborated by Sun Si-miao in China a thousand and more years before.

It is my opinion that TCM acupuncture has lost sight of this story of muscular knots and connective tissue restrictions. In the following pages, I wed Travell's notion of trigger points and concepts derived from osteopathy and physical therapy to the acupuncture protocol I first developed in *Acupuncture Imaging*.[5] In this process, I articulate one possible set of acupuncture treatment strategies. More importantly, I am also attempting to restore a myofascial perspective to acupuncture. Such a perspective is, I believe, capable of transforming acupuncture into a powerful therapy for pain management which can simultaneously restore order to the internal functions of the bodymind.

---

[5] Seem, Mark, *Acupuncture Imaging*, Healing Arts Press, Rochester, VT, 1990

Part I

Treatment Principles

1

A Return to the Body
& the Importance of Touch

When Dr. Janet Travell agreed to lecture on myofascial pain and
trigger point therapy at the Tri-State Institute of Traditional Chinese
Acupuncture, I was elated. This occurred after my colleague, Dr.
Steven Finando and I met for a day with Dr. Travell at her office
and home in Washington, D.C. in the summer of 1991. We had previously sent her a paper we coauthored on segmental release of trigger points based on Oriental physical therapy, acupuncture, and her
own trigger point concepts.

Within minutes of entering Dr. Travell's house, she had taken note
of my short upper arms and other musculoskeletal considerations
and motioned me to a specific chair better designed for my body.
Moments later she asked me to take off my shirt so that she might
show us how she observes, works, and examines for myofascial pain
syndromes. Here was a clinician of the first order intent upon making her points *on and in my body*. The greatest lesson I carried away
from my experience with this remarkable woman was that the key to
pain and its complex dysfunctions is not to be found in the physician's preconceived, objective knowledge but, time and again, in the
very bodies of patients. Dr. Travell returned to the myofascial body,
the body that can be seen, touched, palpated, and manipulated at the
same time that she returned this body to a prominent place in the
practice of medicine.

In May 1992, I introduced Dr. Travell to my students and to numerous other professionals who had come to hear her lecture and watch

her work as a person who had respectfully refused to agree with the beliefs that were commonplace in her time regarding chronic pain and dysfunction. When she had begun her professional career, chronic pain of a nonorganic or non-lesional nature and its concurrent symptoms of distress, such as fatigue, agitation, poor sleep, and vague visceral complaints, were cast outside the realm of medicine and swept under the psychiatric rug. By the end of the nineteenth century, patients who suffered from such ill-defined disorders were considered inappropriate for the modern doctor's waiting room. Space needed to be reserved for the "truly ill," those with organic disease that was potentially serious if not fatal. The diagnosis and cure of organic disease and not the relief of human suffering became the focus of modern clinical medicine. Medical triage was, henceforth, aimed at sorting out patients with lesional disorders requiring medical attention from the far greater number with non-medical complaints which still constitute from 65-80% of a general practitioner's busy practice even today.

However, the problem of what to do with these so-called non-medical complaints and the distressed patients suffering from them remained. If they were sent away with the flimsy reassurance that nothing medical, *i.e.*, organic, was wrong, what were they to do with their suffering? If these signs of distress were not physical problems, what were they, and how could the doctor make a referral that would keep these patients from crowding his busy waiting room?

The answer is now history. A brilliant physician appeared in the right place at the right time with a convenient theory that explained these complaints in psychological rather than physical terms and introduced a new therapy that promised to help these troubled and troublesome patients. That physician was the young neurologist, Sigmund Freud, and, owing to his efforts, this whole set of chronic, nonorganic disorders was rewoven into the fabric of his newly defined psychoneuroses. Henceforth, such complaints came to be diagnosed, more and more, as neurotic, psychogenic, or all in the imagination. The reason, I feel, that medical doctors were so ready to refer such patients to practitioners of this new form of mental therapy and to consider these patients as psychiatric rather than physical cases was because they fit poorly into the newly emerging biophysical and biochemical model of medicine.

By the twentieth century, all medical doctors were trained in the belief that in the absence of organic lesions or systemic disease, recurrent or chronic pain and its associated symptoms of distress were a psychosomatic problem. Its sufferers were hypochondriacs, crocks, and malingerers if they refused to recognize the psychological nature of their distress and insisted upon returning to the medical doctor for follow-ups on their condition.

Freud, in his own study of hysterical neurosis written with Josef Breuer[1], noted that these patients often came with a myriad of complaints, from chronic aches and pains to fatigue, poor sleep, and irritated gut and bowel. He counseled them over and over that these problems were "imaginary" in nature. In a revealing footnote, he clarifies that a neurologist trained as he was to examine the patient's body could not fail to notice physical signs of these complaints and that they often yielded to the twice-daily sessions of prescribed massage and physiotherapy in Breuer's clinic. Follow-up comments on several cases in this study show that, while the psychotherapy carried out by the physician failed, the patients themselves reported obtaining considerable relief from a local physiotherapist! In fact, psychoanalysis has not been shown to help these sorts of chronic discomforts, neither in Freud's case histories nor in those of the psychotherapists who have come after. Most psychotherapists today do not even consider treating patients for such complaints.

Shuffled off to the wrong sort of therapist, patients with chronic pain and dysfunction have suffered in relative silence throughout

---

[1]   Freud, Sigmund and Breuer, Josef, *Studies in Hysteria,* translated by James Strachey, Basic Books, New York, 1987

the better part of the twentieth century. Some quietly visited "fringe" practitioners—chiropractors, homeopaths, osteopaths, and faith healers. But most ended up believing the wisdom of the day, that their problems were all in their heads. Either lie on the psychoanalyst's couch and reveal all or keep a stiff upper lip. Those were the options for far too many sufferers of chronic pain and dysfunction of this sort when Dr. Travell began her work as a physician in the early 1930s.

Dr. Travell refused to go along with these beliefs and this methodology. With her father as an example, a general practitioner who was familiar with some forms of physical medicine and manipulations, and with her own clear proclivity toward taking everything the patient reported totally seriously, Dr. Travell concluded that it was her job to do the medical detective work needed to make sense of the "myofascial jigsaw puzzle" whose bits and pieces were made up of subjective experiences of pain and discomfort.[2]

Therefore, Dr. Travell proceeded at her own pace and to her own rhythm by returning to the body of her patients and believing that right there in the flesh were the answers to the pain that riddled them. It was simply inconceivable to Dr. Travell that these problems were imaginary, and she set about uncovering the physical nature of these aches and pains.

What Dr. Travell discovered were constrictions and tenderness in the soft tissues of the body which often constituted a complex myofascial holding pattern whose origins in repetitive stress and strain had to be unraveled in order to erect a successful treatment plan. A big part of this unraveling was the use of touch as the key to the physical examination. What doctors after Freud had too frequently forgotten and what Dr. Travell has never tired of teaching is the simple art of informed touch as the main means of learning about the true

---

2   Travell, Janet and Simons, David, *Myofascial Pain and Dysfunction: The Trigger Point Manual,* Williams and Wilkins, Baltimore, Volume 1, 1992, p. xi

nature of recurrent aches and pains. This entails entering the realm of the patient's complaints and assuming they have a basis in the physical body. It also means knowing the body well, especially the parts that can be palpated directly.

In restoring the body to its central place in medicine, Dr. Travell also restored touch to its rightful place as chief diagnostic method. The practitioner's hands were thus considered to be the best instruments for such a physical investigation. Finally, Dr. Travell showed how the release of these myofascial constrictions can provide significant relief and often cure of patients' suffering due to chronic, recurrent pain whether through the application of pressure, spray-and-stretch, or trigger point needling.

As an American acupuncturist practicing for some 15 years, I have come to realize that we, too, often function in this gray zone of medicine. The majority of our clients come with recurrent or chronic pain and vague associated signs of distress that have not responded well, if at all, to orthodox biomedicine or to psychotherapy. Acupuncture is often a last resort for such patients.

I now realize that one of the most significant things that I do is to validate the patient's symptoms as real. These symptoms are often uncovered during the examination for tender trigger points, and release of these physical restrictions often provides significant relief from the pain and discomfort. I assumed all acupuncturists worked in a similar fashion and was rudely awakened to the fact that most Western acupuncturists trained according to the TCM model do not undertake a physical examination of their patients at all. This is the same phenomenon that Dr. Travell encountered when she first met with prominent Chinese acupuncturists in the 1970s. They stressed that they knew exactly where to needle without palpating to find the point based on their exact anatomical knowledge of point location.

To my knowledge, in the East only Japanese acupuncturists have retained the classical focus on touching for tender points. In modern Japanese acupuncture as I understand it, palpation is clearly the main diagnostic tool. In the West, French acupuncturists have maintained a focus on the complex meridian system, and the prominent French-Vietnamese physician, Nguyen Van Nghi, has stressed that a large number of complaints are "tendinomuscular" in nature.

I now find that my concerns parallel those of Dr. Travell, and I feel compelled to emphasize to my students and colleagues the need to return informed touch and myofascial palpation to their primary position in diagnosis and treatment if we are to help with pain management. I believe we must follow Dr. Travell in restoring the body of the patient as our central focus. Such therapy is not superficial or symptomatic in such conditions but primary. By releasing the myofascial constrictions and educating the patient in how to prevent becoming constricted again, such problems are often resolved. The bias in TCM acupuncture that assumes most problems to be internal, *zang fu* imbalances requiring treatment directed at the *zang fu* as the primary focus, in my experience, simply does not hold true in the case of recurrent and chronic pain, nor, for that matter, in most instances of nonorganic visceral distress.

It is for this reason that I will dedicate my efforts in this decade to rethinking, practicing, and teaching acupuncture in light of Dr. Travell's perspective. It is my belief that the original Chinese acupuncturists were describing the same subjective experiences as Travell. I believe the Chinese meridian system was an early myofascial map. And further, I believe that freeing up the circulation of qi in the meridians is identical to myofascial release, thus enabling the nervous, arterial, venous, and lymphatic systems to circulate more normally. To me, the famous classical acupuncture dictum that states, "Where there is no free flow, there is pain," is a description of something identical to Dr. Travell's trigger points. Because of this, I believe that tender, *a shi* points are the primary points in the treatment of pain. In this matter, I agree with Bob Flaws when he states:

> [The] dispersal of the *a shi* point often spells the difference between success and failure in the acupuncture treatment of pain. The named and numbered points are theoretically where the qi and blood can best be adjusted. But *a shi* points are the actual location of blockage and stagnation.[3]

To me, unblocking the qi through acupuncture is identical to myofascial release and the meridian pathways are a composite network of potential pathways for the manifestation of pain. I believe the meridian system, articulated over thousands of years of Chinese observation of human suffering and the somatic images these meridians conjure up should guide myofascial investigation and treatment. I also believe that classical acupuncture and modern myofascial perspectives have much to offer each other. My hope in the discussion that follows is to foster such a merger.

---

[3]   Flaws, Bob, *Sticking to the Point,* Blue Poppy Press, Boulder, CO, 1989, p. 109

2

Tender Points Revisited

Classical acupuncture teachings, once again, state that wherever there is pain, there is lack of free flow and that if there is free flow, there is no pain. This is the meaning of *a shi* or tender points in Chinese acupuncture. They are places where there is a lack of healthy, normal free flow.

I believe this simple principle means that, when looking for local points that correspond to a patient's symptoms of pain and dysfunction, acupuncturists must begin by assessing which meridian pathways are involved. Next they should feel along these pathways for tender constricted points. When a patient shouts, "Ouch! You got it!" that is the *a shi* point and that is the point that is needled to disperse the blockage and free up circulation through that area.

In acupuncture discussions, one often hears that so-and-so's teacher advised that the great acupuncturist uses few needles. This is often interpreted to mean that using only one or two needles is the best treatment. But the great French-Vietnamese acupuncturist, Nguyen Van Nghi's interpretation of this classical principle is different. According to Van Nghi, no great acupuncturist uses two points where they can use one. By this he means that, when treating pain, rather than treating the textbook point nearest the patient's pain as well as the actual tender *a shi* point, one should just needle the a shi point itself. According to Van Nghi, the great practitioner trusts his sense of touch and needles only the one point—the tender point found on palpation and confirmed by the patient's subjective response. However, in a complex case, there may be 20 or more of these tender points. In each instance, the great practitioner uses only one point per site, and by that I mean the tender a shi point, not the textbook point.

Because this is contrary to most Western acupuncturists' current practice and in order to appreciate the importance of tender points in the treatment of recurrent and chronic pain, it is necessary to review the notion of tender points from several perspectives or theoretical points of view.

A Shi Points

As stated above, an *a shi* point as described in Chinese acupuncture is any point where, upon palpation, the patient expresses pain and discomfort in response to pressure. *A shi* points are traditionally treated by dispersing needle technique, moxibustion, deep acupressure, cupping, or *gua sha, i.e.*, rubbing with the edge of a ceramic spoon.

Kori

In Japanese acupuncture, *kori* is a general term used to describe areas of bodily stiffness and constriction with discomfort. It stems from modern, so-called scientific acupuncture in Japan. *Kori* is defined as a tight myofascial constriction that may or *may not* elicit discomfort when pressed but which can definitely be felt by the practitioner as a constriction beneath her probing fingers. Some Japanese texts describe over a dozen different shapes and textures for *kori*, all of which constitute different types of myofascial constriction. In Japanese acupuncture, these points are released by direct needling into the dense resistance that signals the presence of *kori*, or by a variety of distal strategies.

Kiiko Matsumoto calls this dense quality of myofascial constriction a "gummy." By this, she means that such constrictions or *kori* feel like an eraser on a pencil. The needle is inserted just until this gummy feeling is contacted. Then the needle is left in place for 10-20 minutes. Sometimes Japanese practitioners use intradermal needles along with or instead of such deeper needling. These intradermals are inserted horizontally just beneath the skin directly over *kori* points and left for three or so days. *Kori* are also treated by application of multiple repetitions of thread moxa directly over their site.

Modern scientific Japanese acupuncture, the style which has dominated Japanese acupuncture for the last 50 years, maintains that, when *kori* are present in the muscles and fascia, they block that area and thus the four circulatory systems of the body are impeded: lymphatic drainage, venous transport, arterial circulation, and nervous conduction. When these systems are blocked, not only will there be pain and discomfort, but the internal regulatory and immune functions will also be compromised. Many Western traditions of massage and deep tissue work, such as Rolfing, speak similarly of the deleterious effect on internal functions of taut constrictions in the muscles and connective tissue, the fabric of life.

Trigger Points

Travell and Simons define a trigger point as a focus of hyper-irritability in a tissue that, when compressed, is locally tender. If it is sufficiently sensitive, such a trigger point may give rise to referred pain and tenderness and sometimes even to referred autonomic phenomena and disturbance of proprioception. Travell and Simons identify several types of trigger points. These include myofascial, cutaneous, fascial, ligamentous, and periosteal trigger points.[1]

---

[1]   Travell, Janet and Simons, David, *Myofascial Pain and Dysfunction: The Trigger Point Manual*, Williams & Wilkins, Baltimore, Volume 1, 1992, p. 4

Travell teaches that virtually all adults harbor many latent trigger points just awaiting activation. These latent constrictions can become activated if a muscle remains in a shortened position for a prolonged period, as when sleeping or during surgery. They may also become activated if the tissue in which they are found is repetitively strained by being held for extended periods of time in the same position, as when typing or cradling a phone to one side. Further, they can also become easily activated when chilled by a cold draft, air conditioning, or the like, especially if the person is fatigued or suffering from postexercise stiffness. These latent tender points can also be activated by a viral illness. This latter fact helps explain many of the aches and pains commonly suffered along with the flu and chronic viral infections, such as chronic fatigue syndrome (CFS) and post-polio syndrome.

When a trigger point becomes active, the body will normally brace against the pain by adopting "guarding habits" that limit motion and ward off the pain. These guarding habits or holding patterns lead to recurrent or chronic episodes of pain that is more dull than acute. This is accompanied by stiffness and generalized dysfunction of the muscles involved. Eventually, such muscles become weakened, even atrophied, and the patient will usually report difficulty with certain movements, such as twisting off a bottle cap or reaching back to fasten a brassiere.

Regarding the relation between classical acupuncture points as depicted in acupuncture textbooks and trigger points, Travell and Simons clarify this point thus:

> Unlike the classical acupuncture points, we do not think of the published TP (trigger point) sites as immutable locations, but as a guide for where to start looking. Every muscle can develop TPS; many muscles have multiple TP locations. Only the most common TP locations are shown in the published illustrations; individual muscles may have TPS in other locations. The TP sites in a given

muscle may vary from person to person; no two people are exactly alike.[2]

If my opinion regarding the flat, classical Chinese acupuncture diagrams is correct, then they were meant, as Travell and Simons' published illustrations are meant, as a *guide to where to start looking*. And if that is correct, then Travell and Simons and their colleagues have rediscovered the same myofascial phenomena discovered by the ancient acupuncturists who made up the first diagrams and descriptions of points and their locations.

What is so startling and important about this is that Travell accomplished this without any knowledge of Chinese acupuncture theory, such as yin and yang, the five phases, or the meridians. Instead, she discovered these phenomena of trigger points based on images of muscles and fascia from Western medicine. If the TCM anatomists had selected these same myofascial images upon which to overlay the classical acupuncture points, I believe they would have arrived at diagrams virtually identical to those in Travell and Simons' texts and articles. They would also have realized that such locations are approximations, not precise portrayals, serving only as starting places for feeling the body's tissues for constrictions.

Modern Japanese practitioners have retained myofascial images from Western anatomy, and it is, therefore, no surprise that their description of *kori* points is very similar to Travell's. According to the Japanese, these points must be touched to be located, and they appear as tightness in soft tissue. The standard TCM descriptions of *a shi* points of which I am aware, on the other hand, include no such discussion of palpable tightness but only discomfort when pressed.

---

2   *Ibid.*, p. 20

Beyond TCM Acupuncture in the PRC

Now that individual exploration and expression is once again permitted in the People's Republic of China, various non-TCM styles of acupuncture are beginning to surface. Examples of such non-TCM styles of Chinese acupuncture are included in *Essentials of Contemporary Chinese Acupuncturists' Clinical Experiences.*

One important example of a non-TCM style of Chinese acupuncture described in this book is based on the clinical experience of Dr. Xi Xiongjiang from the Shanghai College of Traditional Chinese Medicine. According to his experience in treating rheumatoid arthritis, for example, his main points are all local points, and many of these are needled in one session. Further, Dr. Xi describes this disease as a "deficiency in constitution and excess in symptoms." This underscores and corroborates a basic treatment principle of meridian-based acupuncture which we will discuss below.

In Dr. Xi's treatment protocol, one should tonify and support the constitution or root (yin deficiency in the *zang fu*) and disperse the local yang excess in the painful joints. Dr. Xi stresses palpation of the body surface, especially for sensitive and painful points from among the front *mu*, back *shu*, and *Hua Tuo jia ji*. In terms of myofascial anatomy, this means one should search for tender points in the rectus abdominis, erector spinae, and multifidi muscles respectively. He also searches for abnormal manifestations or pain in the following major groups of distal acupuncture points: *yuan* source points, *xi* cleft points, and *luo* connecting points, all of which are on the extremities. While most TCM practitioners select their points by formula and locate them by textbook location, Dr. Xi follows the procedure used by all those practicing what Bob Flaws refers to as an "acupuncturist's acupuncture." Dr. Xi stresses that, "These painful and sensitive spots, subcutaneous nodes, tuberosity and depression of soft tissues, and other abnormal manifestations found in palpation can be used as reference for diagnosis and also used as a basis for acupoint selection."[3]

The most significant exception, perhaps, among modern PRC acupuncturists whose case histories are included in this same anthology is the work of Dr. Guo Xiaozong from the Acupuncture Institute of the China Academy of Traditional Chinese Medicine.[4] Dr. Guo has developed a theory of "effective spots." He classifies these as benign spots, positive spots, and negative spots. Benign spots are spots which, when pressed, relieve symptoms. For example, pressure applied to TB 9 may alleviate migraine. Positive spots are spots where there is pain, chords, and nodules as well as soreness, numbness, skin hypersensitivity, and papules. These indicate that a disease is more superficial or improving. Negative spots are similar to benign spots and are found based on acupuncture meridian distribution theory. Hence, if a positive spot is found at Bl 21, the back *shu* point of the stomach organ, one would search along the stomach meridian itself for a spot, such as St 36, which when pressed relieves the pain at the positive spot or, in this instance, Bl 21. In this case, St 36 is the negative spot.

Dr. Guo states that all three types of points can be found in acute stages of dysfunction. In the remission stage, one usually finds negative and positive spots. The most commonly needled points in this approach are the distal, benign points which relieve local symptoms and negative points which relieve positive tender local points. Dr. Guo feels that effective spots are different from meridian points but underscores their significance in clinical treatment. His procedure is remarkably similar to the Japanese styles taught by Kiiko Matsumoto, where distal points that relieve specific local constric-

---

3   *Essentials of Contemporary Chinese Acupuncturists' Clinical Experiences*, Chen Youbang and Deng Liangyue chief editors; Zhang Kai, chief English editor; Foriegn Languages Press, Beijing, 1989, p. 526-527

4   *Ibid.,* p. 521-523

tions and tenderness are often selected over the local tender spots themselves.

It must be noted here that, as in the local approach to treating tender points, the key is to be sure that the local constrictions—the pain, chords, knots, that is to say, the constrained qi—are deactivated.

Dr. Guo goes on to list seven types of distribution of these effective spots, three based on Western anatomical considerations and four rooted in classical acupuncture point selection methodology. The three anatomical considerations influencing location of these effective spots are:

1. Distribution surrounding branches of blood vessels (LI 4, Lu 3, and Lu 4)

2. Distribution around the neuroplexus and nerve trunk, whence the importance of the paravertebral, *Hua Tuo jia ji* points located in the deep multifidi muscles running along either side of the spine.

3. Distribution in the various muscle groups; for example, throughout the deltoid like Travell's trigger points.

These findings are in keeping both with modern scientific and empirical acupuncture in Japan and with Travell's trigger points.

The four methods of searching for and selecting effective spots are a derivative of the classical acupuncture methods of upper/lower, right/left, front/back, and internal/external. In the classical formulares for selection of effective treatment points, one first looks for points in the lower part of the body to treat problems in the upper body and *vice versa*; for example, treating the back of the knee for pain in the back of the neck and head. French acupuncturists have also taken this method to mean selecting points from the upper/lower greater meridians of the same polarity, *i.e., tai yang, shao yang, yang ming, shao yin, jue yin, and tai yin.* Thus, for instance, one may treat points on the foot *tai yang* bladder meridian for problems on the hand *tai yang* small intestine zone. Specifically according to this approach, one might treat Bl 58 and 59 if tender to relieve scapular pain near SI 10-14.

Next, one looks for points on the right side of the body corresponding to disturbed areas on the left side and *vice versa.* This is based on the notion that, when one side of the body is dysfunctional, the corresponding opposite side will harbor an area of stagnant qi which, when needled, relieves the problem. For instance, one might needle a tender spot near LI 10 on the right side for a case of tennis elbow in the left arm.

The third method for selecting effective points is the method of front/back which dictates that, as in the case of right/left above, one can expect to find effective points that are tender and constricted on the front of the body, directly in front of disturbed areas on the back and *vice versa.* Hence, in chest pain in the pectoralis muscle area near Lu 1 to Sp 20 in an asthmatic, a tender point may be found directly behind this, near Bl 14-43 which, when needled, relieves the chest distress.

Fourth and finally, internal problems of the *zang fu* organs and bowels and qi, blood, and fluids manifest externally along meridians. Palpation along the associated meridian, the lung meridian in the case of bronchitis for example, should yield an effective point, which, when needled, ameliorates the internal disturbance. This internal/external principle is, in my opinion, the supreme acupuncture principle. I believe it substantiates the fact that acupuncture is an external therapy aimed at the surface which can relieve not only external problems but also internal ones.

Dr. Guo interprets these four methods similarly. He looks for symmetrical distribution on the left and right, symmetrical distribution in the upper and lower, crossing and symmetrical distribution, *i.e.,* points that correspond along the same hypothetical longitudes, latitudes, or crossed upper left/lower right correspondences. And finally, he looks for distribution along the meridians. He expects to find points on the same meridian or on the exterior/interior related meridian. For example, points on the liver meridian may be found for problems along the gallbladder meridian and *vice versa*. He also prefers to treat effective points that occur "close to meridian points."

Here I feel he is, to use the obvious pun, simply missing the point. I believe that when an effective point is found by reactivity to palpation, the effective point *is* the point that needs to be needled. If it is near a textbook location of an acupuncture point, I would maintain it *is* the actual point in that instance and to forget the textbook. Japanese point location indications are often given in this fashion and are based on the pragmatic notion that points that need to be needled will be reactive.

Yet another interesting example of a non-TCM understanding of acupuncture point location occurs in the case of Dr. Yu Zhongquan of the Chengdu College of Traditional Chinese Medicine who "thought of using meridians and collaterals as the key links for generalizing (point) indications."[5] This was, I believe, how the pre-TCM classical Chinese texts always listed point indications. French and Japanese acupuncturists have been doing this for the past century.

A final example of tender point thinking in TCM is the work of Dr. He Shuhuai from the Beijing College of Traditional Chinese Medicine, an expert in *a shi* point needling.[6] Dr. He stresses the importance of selecting points based on the location of symptoms, for instance, selecting *tai yang* meridian points for headache at the nape of the neck and occipital region. Regarding acupuncture treatment, Dr. He cites a critical concept in the *Ling Shu or Mirac-*

---

5   *Ibid.,* p. 265

6   *Ibid.,* p. 250-259

ulous Pivot which states that, as he paraphrases, "In acupuncture treatment, it is necessary to examine the excess and deficiency of meridians first, and then touch along the meridians, pressing and snapping them in order to elicit their responses, and then apply the appropriate method of treatment."[7] He continues that, "in order to find out the location of the pain, one should examine the cold and heat sensation and determine the affected meridian."[8]

Needling Tender Points

The above is an especially interesting citation from an undisputedly authentic Chinese acupuncture classic, since snapping palpation is a major palpation technique stressed by Travell herself. Such snapping palpation consists of rolling the taut band of constricted muscle or fascia quickly under the fingertips at the site of the most tenderness, *i.e.*, the trigger points, which often produces a local twitch response (LTR). This is most clearly viewed toward the end of the muscle, close to its attachments.[9]

For years, when I was treating tender *a shi* points based on Van Nghi's protocol for tendinomuscular meridian excess, I noticed that, upon superficial needling or even acupressure at a tender spot, there would be a rippling movement throughout the area. This was explained to me by my teachers as qi moving through the pathway. Only much later did I realize it was a simple twitch in the muscle elicited by contact with the needle!

The superficial needling technique I have developed for needling tender and trigger points, to be explored in detail in Part II, derives

---

[7]   *Ibid.*, p. 252

[8]   *Ibid.*, p. 252

[9]   Travell and Simons, *op. cit.*, Volume 1, p. 60

from this experience and from Van Nghi's superficial tendinomuscular needling of a shi points. I simply locate the tender trigger points according to Travell's methods, trapping them so that I can insert a thin, 34-36 gauge one-inch needle, no more than 1/2 inch in depth in most cases, directly over the trigger points involved. I then insinuate the needle without twirling it, slowly pecking as if trying to spear the point until I feel a dense resistance, Matsumoto's "gummy," beneath the tip of the needle. I stay at the depth where this density increases and the point feels as if trapped and peck steadily in various directions into the dense spot until a twitch response in the muscle or at least a loosening occurs. Sometimes the patient feels the twitch response in the muscle while I feel or see nothing. However, in most cases, I can see it or feel it with the index and middle fingers of my non-needling hand which I place on either side of the point to keep it stationary, pressing down gently with this hand to feel the reactivity of the tissues being treated.

Dr. He underscores the importance of *a shi* points and stresses that they can be located by, a) superficial palpation, feeling for "positive reaction substances," in other words, nodules, chords, etc. that can be palpated, and b) "positive sensations" or subjective local pain, soreness, distension, and numbness on the part of the patient when the points are compressed. According to Dr. He, if palpation does not elicit the point, a point measurement device that detects volume of electrical conductivity can be used. The point with the highest electrical conduction is then regarded as the *a shi* point.

Again there is a fascinating corollary here with Travell's work. Since the Chinese authors cited above continually refer to their reactive and effective point discoveries as new clinical advances, one cannot help wondering if they have recently discovered Travell's work or the tender point Japanese literature. Here is what Travell states in Volume I which appeared a decade ago: "For those who have difficulty in recognizing TPS by palpation, a dermometer, or similar device to measure skin conductance or skin resistance, can be used to explore the skin surface for points of high conductance (low skin resistance), which frequently, but not exclusively, overlie active tps."[10]

The above review of Chinese *a shi*, Japanese *kori*, and Travell's trigger points reveals a great similarity among all three concepts, and it appears that at least a few clinicians in the PRC are returning to this meridian-based acupuncture concept again.

Supporting the Core

Above I have emphasized the treatment of local tender or trigger points as the key missing methodology of modern TCM acupuncture as practiced in the WeSt However, the treatment of such trigger points, while being the *sine qua non* of effective treatment, is not wholly sufficient without appropriate support. I believe that, as Shudo Denmei also maintains, the main theoretical principle beyond the release of local areas of constrained qi in such a meridian-based acupuncture, is contained in an oft-quoted statement by Zhu Dan-xi. Zhu, also known as Zhu Zhen-heng, was one of the four great masters of the Jin-Yuan dynasties. His famous dictum states: "Yang tends toward excess, yin tends toward deficiency."[11]

Japanese practitioners of meridian acupuncture like Shudo Denmei take this to mean that yang corresponds to the meridian system and especially the yang meridians, while yin corresponds to the organs and bowels and their regulatory functions with respect to qi, blood, and fluids. Japanese practitioners working from this theoretical perspective palpate the Chinese pulses at the radial artery feeling for the most deficient pulse for the yin organs/meridians of the lungs, liver, spleen, and kidneys. The heart and heart protector are not assessed or needled in this system. After this is established, the toni-

---

10   *Ibid.,* p. 60

11   Denmei, Shudo, *Japanese Classical Acupuncture: Introduction to Meridian Therapy*, translated by Stephen Brown, eastland Press, Seattle, 1990, p. 108

fication point and sometimes other supportive points are needled for the most deficient yin system detected. Treatment then proceeds with the deactivation of the local yang excess areas, meaning areas of constrained qi.

While this yin deficiency rarely corresponds to the patient's symptoms and complaints and can only be perceived by the practitioner in the pulses, Shudo Denmei clarifies that the yang excess usually does correspond quite closely with the patient's complaints. The areas of constrained qi, in other words, are what the patient experiences subjectively. The tight tender spots found on palpation of a frozen shoulder are the patient's complaint.

Van Nghi, on the other hand, has interpreted this same principle solely in the context of tendinomuscular treatment. He labels the tendinomuscular meridians yang and the regular meridians yin. He then concludes from the above principle that if yang, the tendinomuscular meridian in his interpretation, is excess, then yin, the corresponding regular meridian, must be deficient or tending toward deficiency. He thus advocates dispersing the local tender points along the tendinomuscular meridian pathway involved with superficial needling, while tonifying the tonification point of the regular meridian.

It is now my opinion that Van Nghi's interpretation is erroneous on two counts. First, he singles out the tendinomuscular meridians as the most superficial, hence yang, level, seemingly unaware of the twelve cutaneous regions (*tai yang, shao yang*, etc.) as the most superficial mapping of the meridian system. Secondly, he postulates that the yin deficiency in question refers to the regular meridians. This is in contradiction to Shudo Denmei's interpretation and with it, I believe, most of Oriental medicines' in general that sees the *zang fu* organs and bowels as yin *vis à vis* the meridians as a whole.

While Van Nghi's tendinomuscular treatments are effective for *acute* pain, I have rarely found them sufficient for recurrent and chronic pain disorders. Given his conceptualization, he only treats along a tendinomuscular meridian pathway or its related ones, treating all three yang arm pathways for example. In chronic pain there is often a far more complex myotonic distribution of tender trigger points such that a constriction in the right scapula, for example, may be accompanied by occasional pain and dysfunction in the right, or even more frequently, left or contralateral sacroiliac joint and gluteal muscles of the buttock. Van Nghi's tendinomuscular treatments do not allow for such myofascial compensation and are, therefore, often inadequate for the treatment of recurrent and chronic pain.

Based on these perceived deficiencies in the style in which I was initially trained, and on my own 15 years of clinical and teaching experience, I have, therefore, developed my own protocol for pain management which will be described in Part II. My protocol is similar to that of Shudo Denmei, although I arrived at it before becoming familiar with his work. Such synchronicity with and confirmation by an avowed master of Japanese meridian therapy convinced me that this protocol represents a viable example of a meridian-based acupuncture style of practice. It has proven very useful for me, especially in the treatment of recurrent and chronic pain and is very easy to teach to students and beginning practitioners.

3

Care & Symptomatic Treatment Principles

The acupuncture imaging protocol I have developed has had a number of influences. These include study and translation of French acupuncture texts, especially those of Soulié de Morant, Chamfrault, and Van Nghi; my personal clinical experience; and problems I have encountered in teaching French acupuncture to my American students. Little by little I have come to realize that some of the French acupuncture information is overly intellectualized.

Perfectly clear, absolutely logical French descriptions of treatment of the secondary vessels, for example, seem to me more like pure interpretations of Chinese texts than protocols born of study combined with practice. Several French practitioners I have had the opportunity to observe write far more elegantly than they practice. While I feel the French are definitely on target in focusing their acupuncture on the images of the meridian system and its dynamic interactions, a certain clinical pragmatism seems to me to be lacking. I am especially surprised to find in the French acupuncture literature no critical analysis of what the Chinese concept of qi might really be all about. The French have written of circulating qi without ever questioning what such movement is, where it takes place, and what qi actually refers to. This, it seems to me, results in a certain romanticizing of the concept of qi and with it the whole notion of acupuncture energetics.

It has been my encounter with Kiiko Matsumoto and the Japanese traditions she has taught at my institute that have filled in the gaps in the French approach to acupuncture for me. Kiiko is a consummate pragmatist who teaches interventions based on what works in clinical practice. In Kiiko's teaching, classical acupuncture theory is filtered through a clearly myofascial appreciation of the underpinnings of acupuncture. Rather than engaging in a long intellectual interrogation, like Dr. Travell Kiiko simply rolls up her sleeves and asks the patient to lie on the table so she can begin work. With Kiiko, the physical examination is the evaluation but it is also the beginning of the treatment, and the release of a constricted area is the indication that the treatment is working. Her example and my own clinical work has led me to believe that qi refers, in large part, to the way muscles and connective tissues communicate with each other, become blocked, and are rendered dysfunctional.

This does not necessarily negate the classical concepts or more esoteric interpretations of qi as a vital force. Rather it enhances these by bringing a grounded perspective to bear on the act of needling in naked flesh. While broad systemic changes do occur as a result, or I might say as side effects, of acupuncture treatment, such as increased production of endorphins, hormonal shifts, and the physiological changes that herald the relaxation response, the key, I feel, lies in what happens locally at the site where the needle is inserted. For more discussion of this, the interested reader may see Dick Larson's "The Role of Connective Tissue as the Physical Medium for the Conduction of Healing Energy in Acupuncture and Rolfing" in the *American Journal of Acupuncture*.[1] In this article, Larson quotes Nagahama as referring to acupuncture as "connective tissue therapy."

As I often remark when lecturing on this topic, a perfectly neutral scientist observing practitioners of different styles and traditions of acupuncture would be able to report only one act that they all share in common, namely that each arrives rather quickly at a moment where he or she selects some specific sites and swiftly inserts a few

---

[1]   Larson, Dick, "The Role of Connective Tissue as the Physical Medium for the Conduction of Healing Energy in Acupuncture and Rolfing," *American Journal of Acupuncture*, 1990, Vol. 18, No. 3, p. 257-259

needles into these sites. It all happens in a flash, like a tiny bolt of lightening. It is, therefore, incumbent upon acupuncture students and practitioners to reflect carefully and soberly on what this simple *act of inserting steel into flesh* is all about. In clarifying this issue, I personally advocate reviewing the classical, as opposed to the modern, Chinese TCM acupuncture theories as the French have done. This should be read and interpreted from the vantage point of late 20th century scientific and medical knowledge of the connective tissue, muscles, and fascia as the Japanese are doing.

Such a myofascial interpretation of classical acupuncture energetics leads away from the view of strictly linear pathways that conduct some sort of vague substance or force-like fluid in a pipe to a more variegated image of piezoelectric communication that is carried out at incredible speed throughout the body's tissues. From this myofascial point of view, most beautifully elaborated in Matsumoto and Birch's *Hara Diagnosis: Reflections on the Sea,*[2] we are not so much lifting up barriers to allow a specific substance or force to circulate through channels as we are restoring communication by releasing a tug in the human fabric.

Working Hypotheses

In *Acupuncture Energetics,*[3] I point out something that I find bears repeating often to students and practitioners alike. There are several main filters through which acupuncturists evaluate the data they collect from interviewing, touching, and observing their patients. The main filters are: yin and yang; the five phases; qi, blood, fluids, and spirit; the *zang fu*; and the channels and connecting vessels. I believe that in TCM, the main filters are yin and yang, the *zang fu*, and qi, blood and fluids. Since TCM is based on an herbal, internal

---

[2]   Matsumoto & Birch, *op. cit.*, 1988, especially chapters 7 through 9

[3]   Seem, Mark, *Acupuncture Energetics*, Thorsons Publishers Ltd., Rochester, VT, 1987

medicine perspective, it is focused on the internal *zang fu* functions and what happens to them. Hence, pathological changes are, primarily described as a deficiency of qi or blood, heat in the blood, excess dampness due to spleen deficiency, etc.

In J. R. Worsley's Five Element or what is now becoming known as Learnington Acupuncture (LA), the key filters are essentially identical to TCM but with a twiSt Here, the *zang fu* filter focuses on the psychospiritual aspect of organ and bowel functions which Worsley calls the 12 Officials. The yin/yang filter, on the other hand, is reduced to excess and deficiency in reading the radial pulse, and the qi, blood, fluids, and spirit filter is reduced to qi and spirit or all that is most immaterial. This is in contradistinction, I believe, to modern TCM where this filter is stripped of spirit and pays only lip-service to qi, privileging instead all that is most material, *i.e.*, blood and fluids. While Worsley is clearly biased toward a homeopathic appreciation of pure vibration, TCM is weighted heavily toward a materialist perspective. Worsley, of course, also adds the five phase filter as the key filter for diagnosis and treatment planning, while TCM sees the five phases as a historical curiosity worthy of mention but not terribly relevant clinically.

What is strikingly absent from both the TCM and the Worsley Five Element approaches is the meridian filter which dominates a meridian-based acupuncture style of practice. Meridian-based acupuncture traditions, whether Japanese, Korean, or French, focus first and foremost on the *jing ma*i and *jing luo*—the meridian system as a whole. Secondarily, they focus next in the following order on, a) yin and yang to detect excess and/or deficiency or a hot or cold condition in the meridians themselves, b) five phases in some traditions as the preferred strategy for treating internal root disturbance and imbalance, and c) the *zang fu* or organs and bowels laSt From the qi, blood, fluids, and spirit filter, meridian acupuncture selects qi as the primary focus. Acupuncture thus conceived is an external therapy aimed at restoring and maintaining normal circulation through the meridian system by resolving constrained qi.

French acupuncture, with its detailed investigation of all 71 pathways, has retained the classical acupuncture images, bringing attention to the meridian filter as the main filter for acupuncture therapy. This is in contradistinction to the merely 14 meridians commonly taught in modern TCM, herbalized acupuncture training. Japanese acupuncture brings in a modern, myofascial perspective while at the same time retaining the classical *Nan Jing (Classical Difficulties)* focus on palpation of the abdomen or *hara* and of the acupuncture points themselves as the chief diagnostic method.

In an "acupuncturist's acupuncture," the channels and connecting vessels filter takes precedence over the *zang fu* filter. It is the images of this multilevel and multidirectional meridian system that guide the intake, diagnosis, treatment planning, and placement of needles. From a classical perspective, needles are placed at points of disrupted or constricted qi circulation; while from a modern myofascial perspective, they are inserted into tight subcutaneous or myofascial knots and pulls in the body's fabric. This is done in order to release these surface constrictions and restore normal qi circulation externally and hence internally. In TCM acupuncture, on the other hand, points are needled according to strict textbook locations by means of standardized measurement. These points are also believed to have very specific effects, like herbs, that relate to internal functions. This is not the case in pre-TCM Chinese meridian-based acupuncture nor modern meridian-based approaches where the focus is on correcting meridian blockage and dysfunction with a knowledge that such changes will also improve internal functions indirectly.

It is my belief that, where the treatment of recurrent and chronic pain is concerned, experts from all persuasions agree that there are no truly effective internal medications that work in the long term. Aspirin is too weak and everything else proves too temporary, too addictive, or too mood-altering. I believe the same is true for internal herbal and even homeopathic medicines. I have found that the key in the treatment of chronic and recurrent pain conditions is to manually or through needling release the myofascial holding patterns which are themselves the cause for the development of this pain. In my experience, tender point and meridian-based acupuncture are especially well suited for such myofascial release.

We are now in a position to discuss the issue of root[4] versus local or symptomatic treatment. Various acupuncture styles can be differentiated to a great degree on the basis of their preference for root or for symptomatic treatment. In acupuncture, root treatment usually involves needling the distal points on the lower arms and legs known as the five transport or antique points; while local or symptomatic treatment usually involves needling of points local or in proximity to the site of the pain or pathology. Most styles of acupuncture pay attention to both root and symptomatic treatment. Nevertheless, it is my experience that different schools tend to emphasize one or the other. As with all preferences or biases, it is important and useful to be aware of one's own relative position with respect to others.

---

[4]   In discussing *root* versus *local* or *symptomatic* treatment here, I am not referring to TCM discussion of Root (the underlying cause of a disorder) versus Branch (the effects and symptoms deriving from the underlying cause), but, rather, as in Japanese meridian therapy, to the difference between focusing on treatment of the core or essence of a person's being as opposed to attention to symptoms. While it is more appealing to speak in New Age medicine of treating a person's core or essence, I submit that this is perhaps beyond the capacities of most mortal beings. I would agree that in focusing on a client's symptoms, starting with relief of these symptoms by release of their concomitant constrictions and holding patterns, a practitioner enters into a dialogue with that client's own experience of illness. A meridian acupuncture approach is especially well suited for this direct communication. In the case especially of chronic or recurrent pain, such an approach is deeply effective and long lasting, and capable of transforming a person who has been crippled by pain and dysfunction. Like Shudo Denmei, I never fail to add a core treatment, but the bulk of my work focuses on symptomatic relief and bodymind release.

Core Treatment

The key concept of core treatment is to address treatment to what is believed to be the underlying dysfunction or imbalance expressing itself as overt symptoms. My experience is that in TCM acupuncture, the core or root is virtually always a *zang fu* dysfunction, such as deficient yang of the spleen, rising liver fire, and so on. It should be pointed out that, in TCM acupuncture, almost every patient is given an internal *zang fu* diagnosis each treatment. However, would it not be peculiar if every patient who visited his or her medical doctor left with an internal medical diagnosis? In fact, only 30-35% do, while the rest are reassured that nothing serious is wrong.

TCM acupuncturists should, therefore, not be surprised by the cynicism and distrust some of their patients and many medical doctors exhibit toward these ready internal diagnoses. Why can't a TCM practitioner ever say there is no significant *zang fu* disturbance present? Why must they always affix a *zang fu* diagnostic label to their patients' complaints? And if everyone does, in fact, always have a *zang fu* disturbance, perhaps they do not require treatment unless they become truly dysfunctional. Many ordinary medical doctors will tell many of their patients to just relax and take it easy and stop worrying, while most TCM practitioners, in the United States at least, are more than willing to prescribe an herbal remedy. The readiness to attach a pathological diagnostic label to every human ill is something TCM practitioners might do well to investigate.

Some European acupuncturists who focus on what they perceive to be the core or root see a root imbalance much like a constitutional imbalance. They suggest that root imbalances must be addressed throughout the patient's life regardless of the presenting complaint. According to such practitioners, there is little expectation that the imbalance will be totally corrected. Rather, their intention is to keep this root imbalance within functional boundaries. Worsley's Five Element school uses such a concept which Worsley refers to

as the "causative factor." European approaches have a more constitutional and psychological understanding of this primary imbalance
not dissimilar from homeopathic constitutional remedies. Whether
these interpretations are consistent with classical Chinese acupuncture theory or not, they represent a strong current in certain
European acupuncture traditions and their American derivatives.

A somewhat similar constitutional concept also appears in Japanese
meridian therapy where the root imbalance is assessed from the
radial artery readings for the yin functions of the liver, spleen,
lungs, and kidneys. According to this school of thought, the most
deficient reading indicates the root.

However, no matter whether European or Oriental, the key notion in
root treatment is that the local symptoms that constitute the patient's
complaint are just branches of an underlying imbalance. It is this
underlying imbalance that is the root cause of these symptoms. The
idea, then, is to keep a focus on the root imbalance, while paying
attention to the branches or local symptoms only when acute or pre-
ponderant. For instance, in TCM acupuncture, the root is the focus of
treatment in chronic conditions, while the branches, the local symptoms and complaints, are the focus in acute disorders.

Local Treatment

In TCM acupuncture, branch treatment is largely synonymous with
local treatment. Branch treatment is aimed at the relief of presenting
symptoms and complaints. However, in meridian-based acupuncture
making use of tender point needling, local treatment is root treatment for the treatment of dysfunction in the channels and connecting vessels. Since such local treatment restores normal qi circulation, it can not only alleviate pain but also affect internal disturbances caused by habitual constriction of the qi in the *jing luo*. In
tender point acupuncture, as in Van Nghi's tendinomuscular protocol, it is thought that as much as 65-70% of patients' complaints are

not internal disorders but the result of surface energetic blockages that merely require local treatment to unblock constricted points or areas. In these cases, the core or root of the disorder is in the surface and such local treatment does address this root.

Most practitioners who focus on the treatment of local points—and I definitely place myself in this category—spend the bulk of their time on surface energetic clearing treatments to resolve subcutaneous and myofascial blockages. We rely heavily on release of tender, constricted spots or what I believe is constrained qi which is part and parcel of a chronic pain client's suffering. Nonetheless, most local treatment practitioners also support or tonify the core or root as well. In this sense, the root is not necessarily the root of the imbalance but the underlying energetic layers which are inseparable in both health and disease from the surface. These deeper layers are the core of the superficial circulation of qi and the essence of the person. In this case, knowing what to treat at a deeper level is determined by reading the pulse, palpating the *hara*, or other similar diagnostic evaluations.

It is fascinating to note that the same percentage of patients who are told by a Western medical doctor that they have nothing medically, *i.e.*, organically, wrong may also be told by practitioners of meridian-based acupuncture that they have merely one or more surface, superficial energetic blockages that do not require deeper treatment. My experience is that these are often the same patients with the same conditions. In my experience, the majority of patients told by a medical doctor that they have nothing wrong suffer from nonorganic, non-lesional chronic complaints that are impossible to pinpoint or prove with objective tests. Such problems include chronic fatigue, irritable bowel syndrome, nervous stomach, tension headaches, chronic pain, urinary dysfunction, and a myriad of stress-related disorders.

These complaints represent a large portion of what most acupuncturists treat—people who have been told they have nothing medically wrong or nothing medicine can treat. It is my feeling that the bulk of such patients suffer from what acupuncture calls constrained qi and what Western physical medicine and physical therapy see as myofascial pain and dysfunction. In my clinical experience, local, symptomatic acupuncture—tender point acupuncture—is ideal in such cases.

If we consider Travell's trigger point therapy as a version of local acupuncture when done with dry-needling, or needling without injecting any substance, it is important to note that she and her colleagues have made tremendous advances in the field of chronic pain management. This work is so closely aligned with local acupuncture as to necessitate a close investigation, and the benefits of local acupuncture might well be easier to demonstrate and research if viewed from such a modern, myofascial perspective.

While Travell does not have a notion exactly akin to Chinese root imbalances, she does have a list of internal disorders that she sees as causative. When they are present, they are the focus of treatment, and local myofascial release is merely adjunctive. These causative factors of myofascial dysfunction range from viruses and internal infections to low thyroid and other metabolic imbalances, and nutritional deficiencies.[5] These causative factors are easily uncovered with Western diagnostic tests and can be corrected rather easily in most cases. Travell also lists structural anomalies, such as a small hemipelvis or short leg, as causative factors that have to be corrected with orthopedic lifts and the like. Here again, myofascial work is adjunctive and proceeds poorly if the underlying structural deficit is not corrected.

Travell and her colleagues have proven their success in pain management, and it is both my belief and experience that local acupuncture in particular and meridian-based acupuncture in general benefit greatly from superimposing her myofascial trigger point images

---

[5]   Travell & Simons, *op. cit.*, Volume 1, p. 114-156

over these. In the protocol to be explored in Chapter 10, local treatment is advocated as the focus combined with treatment of deeper energetic layers for support according to French and Japanese acupuncture considerations.

Meridian-based Acupuncture

From a meridian, *jing mai/jing luo* perspective, internal is equated with *zang fu* function and external with meridian functions and pathways. One looks for excesses and deficiencies in the meridian system, expecting excess more often in the yang or the meridians and deficiency in the yin or the *zang fu*. Five phase treatment is reserved in a meridian approach for treating yin deficiency or root imbalance, while local treatment strategies are adopted to treat superficially constrained qi.

In his excellent text on Japanese meridian acupuncture, Shudo Denmei clarifies certain critical terms in Chinese medicine as they relate to an acupuncturist's acupuncture. According to Denmei, five phase acupuncture is the key to root treatment. He goes on to state that internal deficiency is the focus of such root treatment, since internal excess is rarer and harder to diagnose. He begins by stating that yin deficiency, determined by five phases pulse diagnosis, must be tonified using five phase points and strategies. Yin here primarily means the yin organs, the interior of the body, and the blood. Yang, on the other hand, is taken primarily to mean the exterior of the body, the yang meridians, and the qi. Yang excess can be due to an external pathogenic excess, such as wind, cold, and other external stressors, that creates a hyperactive, surface, *wei* protective response or due to the body's compensation for an internal deficiency. In this case, another area of the body increases its activity to take over for the deficient function. Shudo Denmei cites Ikeda, who calls this second type of hyperactive yang, "reactive yang."

This concept is surprisingly close to Hans Selye's concepts of the stress response and his general adaptation syndrome. According to Selye, responsibility for coping with external or internal stressors is shifted to an area best suited to cope with the stress. This thereby compensates for a weak function or system that would otherwise fall under the weight of the attack. This is especially true for chronic, unabated stress, where the organism constantly shifts the burden to areas better able to cope. Typically in my experience, these more "capable" areas are what acupuncture labels the yang meridians and the surface wei level of functioning. Ikeda's concept of reactive yang thus provides a perfect concept with which to talk about the chronic stress disorders so common in our modern times and especially about chronic pain and its associated dysfunctions.

In addition, Shudo Denmei stresses that the yin deficiency underlying such superficial yang excess must be tonified using five phase strategies, while the yang excess (whether pathogenic factor or reactive yang) must be dispersed locally. He also underscores the simplicity of assessing this yin deficiency by palpating the radial pulses for the lungs, spleen, kidneys, and liver. The heart and heart protector, *i.e.*, the pericardium, are not treated in this system. The tonification point for the most deficient yin organ is thus selected as the root treatment. As soon as this is accomplished, the focus and bulk of the treatment turns to dispersal and deactivation of the superficial yang excess.

The assumption that the root or core is typically yin deficient is derived from Zhu Dan-xi, founder of the *Zi Yin Pai* or School of Enriching Yin and his famous dictum that yang is ever excess, while yin tends to be deficient. Shudo Denmei states that, "In meridian therapy the notion that the yin always tends toward deficiency and the yang toward excess is taken to mean that the yin organs and meridians have a tendency to become deficient, and the yang organs and meridians to develop excessive conditions."[6]

---

[6]   Denmai, Shudo, *Japanese Classical Acupuncture,* translated by Stephen Brown, Eastland Press, Seattle, 1990, p. 108p. 108

Shudo Denmei makes some crucial points about root versus local or symptomatic treatment that are fundamental to any meridian-based acupuncture approach. He begins by stating that root treatment is done by identifying the deficient yin pattern, *i.e.*, deficient lungs, spleen, kidneys, or liver. This is corrected by needling five phase points according to five phase principles of tonification. Local treatment is addressed to the symptomatic meridians and areas of the body. In this case, local points in and associated points for that area are selected and dispersed. In other words, treatment begins by tonifying the yin deficiency, and any symptoms that are not thus alleviated are then treated by local, symptomatic treatment.

Denmei admits that, in Japan, there is a large range of diversity of opinion regarding this approach. Some Japanese practitioners of meridian therapy believe that root treatment can alleviate 70-80% of a patient's symptoms, while others state that root treatment is not particularly effective for alleviating local symptoms. In all probability, most Japanese practitioners fall somewhere in between these two extremes. Modern scientifically trained Japanese acupuncturists treat almost exclusively from a local, symptomatic approach, and Shudo Denmei's book was originally, in fact, addressed to them. He is merely asking that they add a tonification point for the yin deficient pattern so that root treatment is not neglected. On the other hand, many of these Japanese scientific acupuncturists accuse meridian therapy practitioners of totally neglecting symptomatic treatment, and Shudo Denmei stresses that this should never be the case. Nevertheless, some practitioners treat only the root for a while, waiting to see if this does alleviate the local symptoms, or, in other words, the constrained qi due to yang hyperactivity and excess. If it does not, they then treat locally as well.

Now where chronic pain and similar dysfunctions are concerned, Shudo Denmei says that root treatment may immediately bring relief, only to have the pain return with a vengeance once the patient leaves the office. And in his case histories in the back of the book, it is clear that Shudo Denmei himself spends more time and more needles on the local aspect of treatment. After all, the root yin deficiency is diagnosed and treated with a couple of points within minutes, while the yang excess demands development of one's own proclivities and style:

> Symptomatic treatment is an area in which every practitioner can display his own talent and unique skills. Each of us must spend a lifetime developing our own treatment style.[7]

This is another characteristic of Japanese acupuncture, namely that practitioners are expected to develop a personal style over time. While root treatment is strictly delineated, *e.g.*, for a lung deficiency, tonify the mother, earth point, Lu 9, and leaves little room for development of a personal style, local symptomatic treatment demands such development. As shown above, even in China, the strictly delineated TCM approach to root or *zang fu* patterns is loosening up and allowing for the development of different styles of acupuncture practice, and this is, it seems to me, precisely in the area of local, symptomatic treatment.

Shudo Denmei makes what may sound like a condescending statement when he says that, although

> . . . root treatment alone may be sufficient to relieve the symptoms, it does not go over so well in Japan to use only a few needles. This is because most Japanese patients equate a larger number of needles with a more thorough treatment.[8]

In the case of recurrent and chronic pain conditions, I believe the patient is correct in demanding more palpation for tender points and more needles because, in my experience, in most instances, the

---

7   *Ibid.*, p. 153

8   *Ibid.*, p. 153

complexity of his or her complaint of pain has been previously glossed over by earlier practitioners. Secondly, most pain patients are acutely aware of where they suffer, and the simple act of validating this suffering by paying clinical attention to these local areas is psychologically astute, is evidence of the practitioner's empathy, and validates the patient's own experience of illness and suffering. So why not spend the extra time and use a few more needles?

Shudo Denmei begins the case history section of his book clarifying that he does not represent the pure Japanese meridian therapy school of practice because he was initially trained in the Sawada school which emphasizes the treatment of tender and indurated points. Shudo Denmei's approach to meridian therapy, therefore, breaks with the Japanese meridian therapy orthodoxy that condones mainly root treatment. In his approach, he combines simple root treatment as delineated above with symptomatic treatment consistent with Japanese scientific acupuncture. Influenced by the Sawada school, Shudo Denmei selects points for symptomatic treatment "less because of their general functions or effects in relation to the diagnosis, than on the basis of differences palpated at the site of the points."[9]

He goes on to clearly and unambiguously state that he prefers to needle the actual spot where there are differences in sensitivity or texture, rather than rely on textbook locations. When he lists points in his case histories, for example SI 10, this should be read to mean the tender or tight point closest to that actual textbook point. He stresses that reactive points are more effective in general and particularly when performing symptomatic treatment. He also adds that indurations or tight, hard constrictions in the tissue always indicate a more chronic reaction than simple tenderness. And he finds that tight areas on the abdomen can be relieved more quickly than similar constriction on the back where more repeated treatments and direct moxibustion prove especially useful. Finally,

_____

9   *Ibid.*, p. 209

again breaking with contemporary Japanese orthodoxy, unless the patient is very fragile or deficient, Denmei prefers to leave the needles in place 10-15 minutes to give the body more time to respond to the needle stimulation.

Suffice it to say that when I first read Shudo Denmei's text, I felt totally at home. Here was a master Japanese practitioner delineating in clear, pragmatic fashion exactly the same principles and approaches that I had developed over a dozen years of practice. These are essentially the same treatment principles that I had developed for myself out of my own clinical experience. I had come to these same conclusions while working against the grain of TCM acupuncture and what I believe is its deleterious effect on the practice of American acupuncture.

I concur wholeheartedly with Miki Shima in his "Getting Acupuncture Education Back on Track: What Our Training Has Been Missing and How We Can Benefit from the Japanese Empirical Schools."[10] In this article, Shima calls for the education of American acupuncturists in basic Japanese pragmatic and empirical approaches. He does so because this style of acupuncture is simply more effective in modern clinical practice the majority of the time.

Levels of Understanding

In my own training in French acupuncture, a key question derived from Chamfrault and Van Nghi's teachings. Was a problem in the surface, *wei* protective energy level, in the internal functional, *ying* or nourishing energy level, or in the core, *jing* or ancestral energy level? I have relabeled this tri-level concept as surface energetics

---

10   Shima, Miki, Getting Acupuncture Education Back on Track: What Our Training Has Been Missing and How We Can Benefit from the Japanese Empirical Schools, *American Journal of Acupuncture,* Vol. 20, No. 1, 1992, p. 33-42

(*wei* level), functional energetics (*ying* level), and core energetics (*jing* level).

Surface Energetics

For me, surface energetics refer to the 12 cutaneous regions, *e.g., tai yang, shao yang*, etc., the secondary vessels, especially the tendino-muscular meridians, and the whole set of activities whereby yang protects yin. At this level, problems are usually due to overwork, excessive activity, overvigilance, hyperactivity, or what modern immunologists call "up-regulation" where the system is working in overdrive. In this layer, we witness the body's holding patterns or repetitively strained zones and tugs in the connective tissue and musculature akin to what Wilhelm Reich termed character armor. Release of these holding patterns is critical not only because it relieves the aches and pains and associated dysfunction generated by local constrictions but also because it frees up the psychological and core energies that are drained in such conditions. This drain or blockage of core and psychological energy can seriously affect both the psyche and soma. While the release of surface constrictions cannot necessarily cure a case of chronic depression in a sufferer of chronic pain, it can ameliorate the psychological condition by liberating the energy that had hitherto been engaged in coping with that actual pain and dysfunction.

Functional Energetics

Functional energetics refer to the level of the *zang fu* organ functions of Chinese medicine as well as to the circulation of yin substances, especially the nourishing or *ying* qi, blood, and body fluids. Visceral disorders are often treated at this level, and it is my experience that TCM acupuncture primarily focuses on this level. Regular meridian treatment strategies are used here, such as source and *luo*, *xi* cleft, transporting points, and *mu* and *shu* points, since the regular meridians or *zheng jing* circulate to the *zang fu* directly.

Core Energetics

Core energetics refer to the *jing* level comprised of prenatal ancestral energies likened by many French authors to the genetic code laid down at conception for the future development of the organism. Acupuncture aimed at treatment of this core level includes eight extraordinary vessel and five phase strategies. Treatment at this level rarely relates directly to the complaints of the patient but rather seeks more generalized harmonization of a preventative as well as constitutional nature.

Chamfrault and Van Nghi have taught that the acupuncturist should begin by assessing which of the three energetic levels—surface, functional, or core—is disturbed. Having ascertained this, he or she should then direct the treatment to the meridians that make up that energetic level. According to Chamfrault and Van Nghi, 65-75% of the problems seen in an ambulatory acupuncture general practice involve the surface or *wei* qi and can be treated by surface tender point release. This can be done either by dispersing the tendinomuscular meridian(s) involved and tonifying the corresponding regular meridians or by simple dispersal of local *a shi* points coupled with stimulation of distal points that have a strong effect on the area under treatment. For instance, LI 4 may be needled distally for head pain. I believe the 12 cutaneous regions must also be envisioned as part of the surface energetic level, especially the six yang pathways that comprise *tai yang, shao yang*, and *yang ming* which tend toward external excess.

In the protocol to be explored in Part II, the focus is on the deactivation of yang excess constriction. The acupuncturist begins by evaluating the three yang greater meridian (cutaneous) regions, palpating all along *tai yang*, the dorsal zone, *shao yang*, the lateral zone, or *yang ming*, the ventral zone as the case warrants. This is based on the location of the symptoms and complaints of the patient. The practitioner feels for tender and constricted knots and bands since these are the signs of constrained qi. These are then deactivated in order to restore normal circulation of qi and myofascial function.

If the patient presents with occipital headache and pain in the upper back and scapula region, the *tai yang* zone is palpated. In this case, the practitioner is looking for tender and constricted points near SI 9-14, Bl 11-14, Bl 40-43, and Bl 10. Treatment of these locally constricted points is then coupled with distal points from the *tai yang*, such as Bl 58-59 and SI 4 and 6 to further disperse this excess. These should also be combined with points to support or tonify *shao yin*, such as Ki 3 and Ht 7, since the *shao yin* may be seen as the yin root of the *tai yang*. Further, the entire *tai yang* zone can be opened and readied for release by treating the extraordinary vessels that energize this zone, namely the *du mai* and *yang qiao mai*, by needling their respective reunion points, SI 3 and Bl 62.

This protocol adheres to classical acupuncture principles as advocated by Shudo Denmei while emphasizing the treatment of tender points for local release and alleviation of symptoms. As stated above, I believe that the latter is crucial in recurrent and chronic pain management. Such a focus on local treatment is not an inferior style of practice as some root practitioners such as Worsley suggeSt In pain management, the validation of a patient's experience achieved by palpation for tender and tight spots is of major therapeutic benefit in and of itself. When these spots are additionally deactivated through acupuncture or what physical medicine refers to as dry-needling, the chronic pain holding patterns begin to yield and therapeutic results increase, often dramatically.

Some people who have attended demonstrations where I show this protocol for treating recurrent and chronic pain, in which as many as 20-30 local needles may be used, have remarked that this is a "hard" style of practice. These critics aver that a "soft" style is always preferable. On the other hand, modern Western medical treatment for recalcitrant pain can be extremely invasive in comparison to such a supposedly "hard" style. Even emg muscle testing is much more invasive than this sort of acupuncture. When I release tender and trigger points, I use very fine, 34-36 gauge filiform needles usually inserted no more than 1/2 to 3/4 of an inch. This is much less invasive than trigger point injection or dry-needling with hypodermic needles. While many points are needled at once, the typical response on the part of my patients is relief that someone is finally tending to all of the areas he or she has experienced as painful for so long. By needling the entire zone of constriction at once, rather than just one or two spots as practitioners of trigger point injection therapy do, it is my experience that one can achieve greater and more lasting release in far fewer sessions.

While it may or may not be accurate to refer to local acupuncture treatment protocols as belonging to a "hard" school or style, what is wrong with an approach that makes rapid progress in complex and recalcitrant pain conditions? It is my belief that, in the treatment of recurrent and chronic pain, any treatment that postpones immediate therapeutic efficacy and avoids local pain relief while attempting a much slower root approach is ultimately a much "harder" style for the patient to bear. To me, such an approach places its ideology rather than the patient's distress firSt The protocol I advocate seeks immediate improvement in quality of life and in the patient's capacity to cope with and enjoy life. In my experience, a prolonged and protracted search for the elusive root without immediately relieving the sites of pain and discomfort is not as efficient and effective as the protocol I am advocating. Nor does such an approach create changes as rapidly in the patient's quality of life.

So-called "soft" styles of acupuncture may superficially appear more compassionate since they involve less needle insertions per treatment. But since their treatments are not as effective, where is their ultimate wisdom and compassion? Therefore, in my opinion, such indirect and minimalist approaches offer little to the main stream management of pain. This is all the more ironic since most Westerners, patients and practitioners alike, associate acupuncture primarily with the relief of pain.

4

Myofascial Chains

In her discussion of myofascial chains in the low back and legs in chronic low back pain sufferers, B. J. Headley extends the discussion of trigger points beyond the concept of local neural hyperirritability at such points.[1] Physical therapists with special interest and training in myofascial release of trigger points are often frustrated by the arduous nature of ischemic compression, spray-and-stretch, and other such techniques for the release of trigger points in complex myofascial pain syndromes and by the appearance of trigger points in other areas of the body following release of points localized in the initial target zone. Referring these patients for acupuncture or trigger point injection has proved equally frustrating for physiatrists. In too many instances, local release is achieved while the problem becomes aggravated elsewhere.

What is so interesting about Headley's discovery of entire myofascial chains—strings of related trigger points or zones—is that these chains appear very similar to acupuncture pathways. I have come to the conclusion after many years of teaching and practice that acupuncture points refer to general potential sites in the myofascial territory that are *predisposed to dysfunction concomitantly*.

In other words, acupuncture points and pathways provide a means of

---

[1]   Headley, B. J., EMG and Myofascial Pain, *Clinical Management,* Vol. 10, No. 4, July/ August 1990, p. 43-46. This is a reworked version of an article that originally appeared with Steven Finando in *Advances Magazine* for physical therapists.

imaging myofascial pain and dysfunction. For instance, Headley discovered a myofascial chain in the lower extremities during her study of 19 back patients. This chain was identified after extensive static and dynamic emg evaluation, four-channel dysregulation, and comprehensive soft-tissue evaluation for trigger points and referred pain patterns. It extended from the piriformis and anterior pectineus, through the tensor fascia lata and biceps femoris, and down to the gastrocnemius and soleus. The trajectory of this myofascial chain corresponds exactly to the low back and lower extremity segments of the dorsal and lateral zones, *i.e.*, the bladder and gallbladder pathways of acupuncture.

As discussed above, it is my experience that most American acupuncturists no longer treat tender or tight spots and, hence, never really achieve myofascial release in their recurrent and chronic pain patients. In the case of trigger point injection, there are two problems that frequently arise. First, the use of anesthetics, such as Procaine and Lidocaine, has been shown to have harmful side effects in some cases. Researchers have found that comparable results can be achieved with any number of substances, such as saline solution, benzyl salicylate, camphor, or by the use of dry-needling with no substance injected.[2, 3, 4] Secondly, such injections use thick, hollow hypodermic needles. These are quite painful and can cause damage to the blood vessels. Therefore, typically these are inserted into only one or two local trigger points per session. They are never inserted along an entire zone of pain and its referred myofascial chain.

[2]   Baldry, P. E., *Acupuncture, Trigger Points and Musculoskeletal Pain,* New York, Churchill Livingston, Inc., 1989

[3]   Lewit, K., "The Needle Effect in the Relief of Myofascial Pain," *Pain,* 1979, 6: 83-90

[4]   Martin, A. J., "Nature and Treatment of Fibrositis," *Archives of Physical Medicine,* 1952, 33: 409-413

Most American acupuncturists, on the other hand, treat the entire chain or acupuncture meridian. However, in my opinion, they rarely discover or deactivate the actual trigger points in this chain. The physician or osteopath who does locate with great precision the primary trigger points for a given disorder often ignores the secondary trigger points in the distal, related myofascial chains.

After 15 years of practicing acupuncture, I have come to the conclusion that reactive points are far more effective than textbook points for chronic pain management. In discovering the concept of trigger point deactivation, I have realized that my own experience confirms what has already been so well documented and argued by Travell and Simons. In his informative textbook on this subject, British physician, P. E. Baldry, discusses the same notion. Dry-needling into trigger points, in his case with solid acupuncture or emg needles and based on Western myofascial understandings rather than on Chinese metaphysical concepts, yields highly effective treatment of myofascial pain disorders with immediate applicability in mainstream medicine and health care.

While Baldry's goal is to interest medical doctors in this acupuncture/dry-needle approach, he fails to take into account the fact that very few doctors are trained to palpate for trigger points. Fewer still have the time or inclination to do so. Even osteopaths, whose training generally includes these skills, are abandoning palpatory therapies in favor of more orthodox medical techniques and procedures. Baldry doubtlessly hopes that medical acupuncturists will also try out his myofascial approach. However, in my experience, few acupuncturists except the Japanese are so inclined or prepared by their training to do so.

 In tender point acupuncture as I have come to practice it, it is not necessary in the soft tissue evaluation to distinguish between primary, secondary, and satellite trigger points as Travell and Simons do. In my own practice, I search for chains of reactive points in the dorsal, the lateral, and the ventral zones as explored and discussed in Part II. These points are all deactivated by acupuncture/dry needle insertion until a characteristic twitch response or fasciculation is achieved. As discussed above, this response indicates release of muscle spasm and constriction.

While one might say that Headley's EMG biofeedback and soft tissue evaluation for trigger point zones and chains is a mere recapitulation of concepts established by Chinese acupuncture thousands of years ago, I feel this is exactly the research necessary to demonstrate to Western myofascial practitioners the beauty and power of the simple Oriental physical therapy and acupuncture concept of evaluating and treating upper/lower, right/left, front/back, and external/internal myofascial chains. In other words, in my experience, there is always an entire myofascial chain, such as the one discovered by Headley for low back pain patients, in any complex or chronic pain case. These chains predominate in one or more of the major zones—the dorsal, lateral, and/or ventral zones.

I believe dry-needling of the entire zone, not just a few points as most trigger point injection and orthodox acupuncture treatments do, is far more effective for such conditions than any current physical therapy technique, TCM acupuncture, or trigger point injection therapy. Such an approach to chronic pain management can be easily integrated into mainstream pain management protocols for the immediate benefit of the pain sufferers themselves.

5

Somatovisceral & Viscerosomatic Pain & Dysfunction: Organs, Meridians, or Both?

A point I impress upon my acupuncture students regarding the intake and evaluation process is the need to assess whether a problem is in the internal, *zang fu* functions, the external, meridian systems, or both.

When I wrote *Acupuncture Energetics*,[1] my goal was to restore communication between the two major acupuncture styles in the United States at the time, TCM or eight principle acupuncture and Five Element acupuncture according to J. R. Worsley. While I knew from my French training and from experience that the majority of problems are external, meridian problems, the case histories in the back of that book focused solely on internal, *zang fu* problems. My intention was to show these two schools of thought that they are actually closer than they think to each other. However, in so doing, I played down the importance of a meridian perspective to acupuncture. In this sense, I had fallen into the same trap as most English-speaking acupuncturists in the 1980s. I was speaking a TCM acupuncture language. I was talking about acupuncture from an internal, *zang fu* perspective as opposed to a meridian-based perspective.

---

1   Seem, Mark, *Acupuncture Energetics*, Thorsons Publishers Ltd., London, 1987

My last book, *Acupuncture Imaging,*[2] was written to correct the mistaken assumption that most problems are internal, *zang fu* problems. In fact, my experience suggests just the opposite. I believe that, from an acupuncturist's point of view, most disorders are more accurately described as meridian, surface energetic blockages than as internal, organ functional ones. If I were to write case histories from my actual clinical experience rather than tailoring them to match TCM patterns of disharmony, one would find that easily 60–80% of these could be characterized and treated as meridian problems.

It is the internal, herbalized, TCM perspective that assumes most disorders are *zang fu* problems. While TCM has clearly articulated and fully elaborated *zang fu* patterns, I believe that most classical Oriental acupuncture traditions and, most notably, Japanese meridian therapy limit categorization of zang fu, internal disorders to simple patterns of excess and deficiency and sometimes heat and cold in the yin organ functions. Shudo Denmei's methodology is a case in point. In his admittedly somewhat unorthodox approach to meridian therapy, he simply evaluates quickly for deficiency in the spleen, liver, lungs, or kidneys. He then tonifies the weakest *zang* by way of its related tonification point on the regular meridian in question. The remainder of the treatment is focused on the careful identification and release of tender points with attendant relief of symptoms by deconstraining areas of blocked qi.

When I first began stressing to my students the importance of determining whether a problem was in the internal *zang fu*, the external meridians, or both, the Japanese texts currently available in English had not yet appeared. At that time, my ideas were met with cynicism by many practitioners trained in TCM. These practitioners typically wanted to know where diagnosis of meridian problems was even discussed in the English literature derived from China, let alone practiced. I was teaching from my own translations of French

---

2   Seem, Mark, *Acupuncture Imaging*, Healing Arts Press, Rochester, VT, 1990

authors, primarily Soulié de Morant, Van Nghi, Chamfrault, and Schatz. Royston Low's excellent summary of the secondary vessels[3] was not yet available. To this day, the work of most of the French authors cited above is not available in English. When my faculty members went to do postgraduate training in the PRC, in most cases they returned even more convinced that real (read, TCM) acupuncture is *zang fu* acupuncture. Some even advocated that the institute should devote far more time to teaching TCM pattern differentiation and treatment and far less, if any time, to French and Japanese meridian acupuncture. It was difficult to maintain a meridian per-spective in those days when everyone else was swept up by the political correctness of TCM.

Happily now, the balance seems to be shifting. There are several books available on Japanese acupuncture and at least some of the French is also available. The excellent acupuncture training program for physicians developed by Dr. Joseph Helms for the office of Continuing Medical Education of the UCLA school of medicine is also based on French meridian acupuncture, and his graduates fare quite well with this approach in a wide range of health care prob-lems. Blue Poppy Press has made a major contribution to acupunc-ture in the West by publishing pre-TCM and non-TCM acupuncture texts deliberately to demonstrate the diversity of traditions and styles that constitute the richness of acupuncture. Even in the PRC, as we have seen above, there are those who are now practicing non-*zang fu* styles of acupuncture that focus on meridians and tender points.

It is clear to me that, from its inception till relatively recently, acupuncture has focused on the stuff of acupuncture, namely the free flow of qi through the meridian system. Chinese herbal medi-cine, on the other hand, focuses on the functions of the internal organ and on the humors or blood and fluids that circulate internal-ly. While Western practitioners of TCM have adopted this latter, herbalized perspective and in their clinical practice usually combine

---

3   Low, Royston, *Secondary Vessels of Acupuncture,* Thorsons Publishers Ltd., London, 1983

acupuncture with the prescription of herbal medicine, French and Japanese acupuncturists have tended to retain a far more classical focus on the meridian systems and the way in which blockages occur therein. Given my own training in French acupuncture and the great impact that Kiiko Matsumoto has had on me and my institute, it is not surprising that I would develop yet another perspective on a meridian-based style of practice.

Feedback from readers of *Acupuncture Imaging* has confirmed for me that this protocol for practicing a meridian-based acupuncture is consistent with classical Chinese meridian-based acupuncture and modern Japanese meridian therapy. I have also learned along the way that modern scientific or medical acupuncture in Japan works from a decidedly myofascial perspective. In many respects it is very similar to Travell's trigger point myofascial work with which the modern Japanese are quite familiar. The integration of Travell's theory and practice into a meridian-based protocol is, therefore, consistent with the development of acupuncture in Japan over the past 50 years. While there is much difference of opinion in Japan between the classically rooted, meridian therapy tradition and the modern scientific, symptomatic approach, I believe this difference is simply one of emphasis. Some practitioners emphasize treating what they consider to be root disorders, while others focus primarily on local treatment. However, it is my opinion that it is the combination of both styles together, similar to Shudo Denmei, that taps the essence of classical acupuncture in all its breadth. As in so many other spheres, the Japanese here again show their facility for combining the insights of their classical heritage with those of modern science.

An interesting historical fact regarding TCM acupuncture textbooks is in order here. None of the first English language acupuncture textbooks from the PRC mentioned the secondary vessels let alone depicted them. They listed only the 12 regular meridians plus the *ren mai and du mai*. However, acupuncture texts from the prc began to include illustrations of the secondary vessels shortly after two major visits to China by Van Nghi himself. While there, he gave the

Chinese copies of his celebrated texts. Royston Low's book on the secondary vessels had also appeared by that time. It is, therefore, quite possible that curious French and English-speaking acupuncturists in the PRC went back to their own literature on the meridian systems for confirmation of their importance. While the description of the secondary vessels in most English language TCM texts stops there with no further discussion of how to treat using them, it is clear from firsthand reports of students returning from study in China and from the many descriptions of meridian-based styles in *Essentials of Contemporary Chinese Acupuncturists' Clinical Experiences* reporting on work begun in the mid–1980s, that there are proponents of meridian-based styles of acupuncture alive and working in the PRC.

While those practitioners included in *Essentials of Contemporary Chinese Acupuncturists' Clinical Experiences* are all quick to state that their discoveries are new, I cannot help wondering if we are witnessing various family styles coming out of the closet now that free expression has become more possible. It is also likely that some of these researchers are familiar with the Japanese literature since medical study exchanges are beginning to bridge these two cultures. As people begin to really break free of the deleterious effects of the Cultural Revolution in the PRC, acupuncture practitioners seem to be following suit. There are now many voices in China speaking of different approaches, sometimes combined with herbs, sometimes combined with *qi gong*, sometimes practiced alone, which extend beyond the narrow confines of TCM acupuncture as transmitted to the West in the early 1980s.

In brief then, while TCM-trained practitioners might have some difficulty responding to the question of whether a problem is in the *zang fu*, the meridians, or both, this critical question receives a consistent reply from meridian-based acupuncturists. For us, problems are most often seen as lying in the surface energetic, external zones where constrained qi causes a myriad of tight, tender spots. The focus of practitioners such as myself is on freeing up the surface by clearing these meridian blockages. Those of us who stress local treatment tend to treat many local points to directly free up the local knots and bands of constrained qi.

In my experience with chronic pain patients, I find this approach works beSt Partially this is because attention to local tender points validates the patient's own experience of illness. Such validation alone is a powerful tool in pain management when so many patients have been told their suffering is all in their head. Once the surface is freed or while freeing it, meridian-based acupuncturists also support or tonify the root or yin deficiency imbalance. This may be equivalent to an imbalance detected on the *hara* or abdomen, an imbalance detected on the radial pulses, an extraordinary vessel, or a five phase imbalance. There are various interpretations of the core or root, and, in chronic conditions, a TCM *zang fu* pattern may also be considered. One can easily tonify deficient yang of the spleen as the root aspect of a treatment instead of using five phase strategies to tonify spleen earth in a meridian protocol.

Modern scientific acupuncturists constitute the majority of practitioners in Japan today. In his book written for this audience, Shudo Denmei represents the minority meridian therapy school of thought when he urges a return to the classics and to a focus on five phase tonification strategies to correct root imbalance. These modern Japanese practitioners are already well versed in local treatment since it is the focus of their approach. For example, they all know how to treat the quadratus lumborum and iliocostalis muscles in low back sufferers and have various local and distal strategies for such myofascial acupuncture release. Shudo Denmei simply wants to encourage this group to add root support in order to deepen and prolong the therapeutic effects of treatment.

In a way, I am attempting the opposite. I believe that most of my Western colleagues, unlike the Japanese myofascially-oriented acupuncturists, are either root practitioners of the Worsleyan Five Element tradition or TCM *zang fu* practitioners. In either case, it seems to me that both are focused on internal harmonization. I would like to encourage both these groups to return to the classical knowledge of the meridian system, to try out meridian strategies, and to investigate the issue of *a shi*, tender point treatment from Travell's trigger point perspective. I believe that if they do this, they will find that, especially when treating chronic and recurrent pain and dysfunction, they have a far larger and more effective clinical armamentarium with which to combat these difficult problems. I also believe that the inclusion of such local treatment will in no way hinder or detract from their internal regulation. They may still want to use front *mu* and back *shu* points for the *zang fu* or Officials that are disturbed, and perhaps they will also prescribe herbal remedies for this aspect of their patients' disorders. But the local release of tight, tender points will be their powerful trump card, providing a physical medicine focus for their treatment of complex pain patterns. Combined with informed referrals to specialists in physical medicine and rehabilitation, physiatrists, osteopaths, physical therapists, chiropractors, and bodyworkers, they will have a successful pain management program to offer their patients.

It should now be clear that, in order to answer the question, "Is the problem in the *zang fu* organs, the meridians, or both?", we first need to know the bias or leaning of the acupuncturist being queried. If the practitioner is from a root school of thought, the answer will usually be the *zang fu*/Officials. If the practitioner is from a local treatment orientation, then the meridians will be the focus. But in either case, the other perspective should not be neglected. Local treatment benefits greatly from root support, and root treatment is greatly enhanced when meridian blockages are cleared.

Organic or Functional Disturbances?

Interestingly, this question has a long history in Western medical discussion as well. As described above, debate raged throughout the nineteenth century in European medical circles as to whether nonorganic, non-lesional disorders should be considered a part of medicine and included in medical education and practice.[4] Most prominent physicians and researchers advocated casting those with such disorders out of the busy general practitioner's waiting room so that he might get on with curing those things medicine was truly about: infections, epidemics, organic disease, damaged viscera, or musculoskeletal defects.

Others argued that these non-lesional, nonorganic disorders, often referred to, then as now, as functional, were at the very heart of medicine and such complaints were precisely the things for which most patients consulted a physician.[5] Even the least "organic" of the lot, chronic fatigue, deserved a central place in medical education and clinical practice. These practitioners argued that even though a disorder is not organic or visceral, the problem is still somatic and requires somatic intervention. They recommended hydrotherapy and massage to improve circulation and to clear away congested blood and lymph fluid, a nourishing diet, and rest and relaxation combined with tonic exercise, such as a brisk daily walk.

Unfortunately, those arguing to include functional disorders within medicine lost at the turn of the century and, in short order, fatigue disappeared as an acceptable medical diagnosis. With it went the whole vitalist notion of human energy. By the 1930s, neurasthenia, the late nineteenth century's genteel name for fatigue, was rarely if ever discussed in medical circles. Freudian psychology had helped to recast these unwanted disorders as psychiatric, not medical, problems. Some of these disorders were classified as frankly psychological and imaginary and others as psychosomatic. The word *functional* today is still often used by physicians to mean psychosomatic.

---

[4]   Foucault, Michel, *The Birth of the Clinic: An Archeology of Medical Perception,* Vintage Books, New York, 1975, p. 88-90; 160-163

[5]   de Fleury, Maurice, *Les Grands Symptomes Neurastheniques,* Felix Alcan editor, Paris, 1901, especially chapter XI

As stated in the preface and in Chapter 1, Travell began her career in medicine surrounded by this psychosomatic atmosphere. She should have understood most of her chronic pain patients to be suffering from psychosomatic, functional disorders, that is to say, from primarily nonphysical, non-somatic problems in nature and origin. But she disagreed so fundamentally with this notion that she ignored the entire psychosomatic interpretation of such problems and dedicated the next 60 years of her life to showing just how physical and somatic these problems really are. The entire field of physical medicine and rehabilitation would never have flourished as it has if it had not been for Travell's refusal to see myofascial pain as psychosomatic.

Dr. Travell discusses this issue of functional problems with visceral symptomatology and visceral disease with functional and somatic symptoms under the rubric "somatovisceral versus viscerosomatic pain and dysfunction," thus addressing in different language the acupuncture question regarding *zang fu* organ versus meridian problems and the larger medical debate over functional versus organic disorders.

Somatovisceral Pain & Dysfunction

The issue of somatovisceral and viscerosomatic effects is primarily addressed by Travell and Simons in Chapters 42 and 49 of Volume I in which muscular constriction and pain in the front of the torso is discussed.[6] It should be pointed out that physicians tend to expect pain in the back of the body to be musculoskeletal, while they expect pain in the front of the body to be visceral and organic. Physical examination of the front of the torso is, therefore, done to rule out organic disease or other visceral disturbance. Laboratory and other screening tests are often ordered to confirm or rule out a visceral diagnosis.

---

6   Travell & Simons, *op. cit.*, p. 585-586; 672-674

However, if the patient's chief complaint is recurrent or chronic pain and dysfunction in the front of the body, and physical palpation over the organs as well as laboratory and other tests all fail to detect anything organic or lesional, the patient's pain is typically considered psychosomatic in nature. This is especially true if there are some vague and non-alarming visceral symptoms like diarrhea, intestinal gas and bloating, fatigue, frequent urination, and the like. It is rare for physicians to take such pain and dysfunction seriously after their examinations and tests all show up negative. It is even rarer for physicians to go ahead and touch the area where the patient experiences pain, feeling the soft tissue, muscle, and fascia for signs to explain this localized discomfort. As mentioned above, chronic pain of this sort, even when associated with some minor visceral complaints, is considered to be outside the realm of physical medicine by most physicians. In my experience, most TCM-trained acupuncturists also fail to palpate the body surface in such chronic conditions, diagnosing instead internal *zang fu* organ dysfunction.

Dr. Travell, on the other hand, advocates taking the pain quite seriously, so seriously as to warrant a physical examination. In such cases, palpation of soft tissue often reveals the presence of exquisitely tender trigger points. Once these points are inactivated, the visceral complaints disappear or significantly lessen. This is what Travell and Simons refer to as somatovisceral effects. Somatovisceral effects occur in cases where a myofascial disorder leads to disturbance of the viscera. In such cases, resolution of the myofascial disorder relieves or eradicates the visceral symptoms, and no internal visceral treatment is required. Dr. Travell cites some fascinating examples of this.

For instance, a somatovisceral effect in the chest arises in the presence of trigger points in the right pectoralis major muscle halfway between the sternum and the mammillary line between the fifth and sixth ribs or roughly the area of Ki 22 in acupuncture. This trigger point can cause paroxysmal arrhythmia, and deactivation of the trigger points has been shown to eradicate this arrhythmia.

Another example may be found in the abdomen where there are sometimes trigger points in the rectus abdominis and internal and external oblique muscles. Interestingly, this is the same area in which are found the front *mu* points associated with *zang fu* organ dysfunction in acupuncture. Travell and Simons point out that trigger points here often cause visceral disturbances such as diarrhea, vomiting, bloating, colic in children, burping, dysmenorrhea, food intolerance, bladder pain, residual urine and dribbling urination, flatulence, inability to pull in the stomach, and pain over the gallbladder or at McBurney's appendicitis spot. Trigger point activity in the skin or subcutaneous trigger points of the lower abdomen, as well as trigger points in the muscles of the lower abdomen, can cause urinary frequency, urinary urgency, and kidney pain, as can trigger points in old appendectomy scars.

Practitioners of European scar therapy similarly report visceral disturbance throughout the abdominal and pelvic area to be caused by the adhesions in old scars and use a technique akin to Travell's injecting Lidocaine into the subcutaneous scar tissue itself. I had one such patient, who suffered for years from a terrible case of what physicians had diagnosed as colitis. Acupuncture treatment led to no improvement whatsoever. Dr. Yves Requena, a noted French medical doctor and acupuncturist who was giving a seminar at our institute, agreed to see this patient in grand rounds. Requena pointed out a huge scar from a five year-old gallbladder surgery and told the participants present about German scar therapy. He taught a physician present how to do Lidocaine injections into the scar, and, after only a few injections over two weeks, the patient's colitis totally disappeared.

I had another patient with numerous scars from surgeries to reconstruct the urethra and bladder who had incredibly tender trigger points in the rectus abdominis muscles right above the pubic bone bilaterally. This patient's main complaint was frequent urination and dulled sexual functioning attributed to hypochondria by the surgeons. I treated the rectus trigger points as well as a few tender spots directly in the scars, and the patient's urinary and sexual symptoms virtually disappeared within a few days.

Acupuncturists see many such somatovisceral disorders, and, to our credit, we take such disorders seriously. However, TCM-trained practitioners rarely palpate the actual area of discomfort and would, therefore, do well to heed Travell's advice. Physical examination is critical in such cases, after medical screening has been done to rule out infection or organic disease that might be beyond the acupuncturist's scope. Such palpation often reveals trigger points that, when released, relieve the visceral complaints as well.

Viscerosomatic Pain & Dysfunction

Viscerosomatic effects, on the other hand, are the result of visceral disease which cause the formation of somatic trigger points. These trigger points and their associated pain and dysfunction often remain after the visceral disease has been resolved. In such cases, deactivation of the trigger points provides great and often decisive relief almost immediately. Acupuncture tender point therapy is, therefore, also indicated in such cases. In that instance, it is used not to treat the visceral disease *per se* but to relieve the associated complaints and discomfort. However, practitioners should be forewarned that relief of discomfort does not necessarily mean the eradication of the visceral disease. Therefore, such patients should only be treated by acupuncture if also under the care of a physician who can properly monitor the visceral condition.

Coronary insufficiency or any other intrathoracic disease that refers pain from these viscera to the anterior chest wall are examples of conditions which can perpetuate trigger points and pain. Such conditions can cause the activation of satellite trigger points in the pectoral muscles. In such cases, deactivation of these trigger points eases this discomfort but does not change the visceral disease itself. Yet another example is reflex spasm and rigidity of the abdominal muscles in response to acute appendicitis. Trigger points are often found upon palpation to be present in such spasmed muscles.

Likewise, duodenal ulcers have been found to cause trigger points in the abdominal muscles over the duodenum. Typically, pain from these ulcers initially responds well to medication. However, they also tend to become unresponsive to medication until and unless these trigger points are deactivated. At that point, the medication again works well, and the combination of tender point acupuncture and medication for such chronic ulcers is well indicated. The same situation occurs in the case of peptic ulcers, intestinal parasites, acute internal trauma, and/or chronic occupational or repetitive strain. All of these may perpetuate trigger points, and their release can prove of great relief. Nonetheless, the underlying medical condition must still be addressed.

There are other nonorganic disorders of a chronic nature that also fall under the viscerosomatic category. These include trigger points in scars; stress disorders pushing the sympathetic system into overdrive with resultant disorders of the sympathetic and parasympathetic organ functions coupled with severe fatigue; emotional tension; prolonged exposure to cold as in the case of a butcher working in a refrigerated meat locker; viral infections; poor posture; and such structural inadequacies as a shortened leg or a small hemipelvis. All such cases can be helped by release of the trigger points in the areas of discomfort and dysfunction, but relief will not be lasting unless the internal visceral, structural, or other problem has been addressed. Usually this requires appropriate medical treatment or at least supervision. It is for this reason that I require all my patients with recurrent or chronic complaints to consult a physician, and I have developed a network of generalists and specialists upon whom I can call.

Travell and Simons' discussion of somatovisceral and viscerosomatic effects points out the importance of palpation whenever the patient reports pain and associated dysfunction, even when nothing medical, *i.e.*, organic or lesional, can be detected. Acupuncturists working from a myofascial perspective will often detect tender points that account for the patient's symptoms, just as do Travell and her colleagues. This can only help to bring acupuncture into the mainstream, multidisciplinary treatment and management of pain.

Because of the importance and efficacy of working from such a myofascial perspective when treating with acupuncture, I keep both volumes of Travell and Simons' *Myofascial Pain & Dysfunction: The Trigger Point Manual* on my consultation desk and refer to them constantly. I often use them to show clients Dr. Travell's images of myofascial distress which often match their own symptoms exactly. I also often show my patients which meridian pathway is involved. Typically, this parallels Dr. Travell's images. My encounter with Dr. Travell's trigger points has enabled me to clarify my work as a local treatment, meridian-based acupuncturist, and this has resulted in greatly enhancing the efficacy of my treatment of recurrent and chronic pain disorders. Trigger points, *kori*, and *a shi* points are powerful phenomena that can and should guide our palpation and keep us grounded in a direct relationship with the body of the patient before us. Such palpation clearly demonstrates that the overwhelming majority of patients' seemingly subjective experience of pain and dysfunction is actually based on the objective and easily demonstrable presence of myofascial knots and bands. This is something any practitioner can experience who is willing to make the effort and spend the time *touching* the person whose discomfort they hope to alleviate.

Part II

Treatment Protocols

6

A Tender Point Acupuncture Protocol for Pain Management

To sum up the treatment principles enunciated in previous chapters, which for me comprise the working principles of tender point, meridian-based acupuncture, we must begin with the principle that yang tends toward excess and yin toward deficiency. In the context of a meridian-based acupuncture, this yang excess should be understood as hyperactivity and up-regulation in the surface energetic zones. This results in a multiplicity of cutaneous and myofascial constrictions in the involved zones. These constrictions are variously called *a shi, kori,* and trigger points. In this style of treatment, these yang excesses are dispersed and deactivated locally. Distant or non-local points from the same meridians involved in the affected zone are also used to aid in dispersal of this yang excess at the same time that points are needled to support yin. Such distant points are selected based on the following principles:

Upper/lower

This means that points on the lower body are selected to treat disorders of the upper body and *vice versa.*

Left/right

This means that points on the left are used to treat a disorder on the right and *vice versa.*

Front/back

This means that points directly in front of the disturbed area on the back are used to treat that area and *vice versa.*

Internal/external

This refers to the release of external constrictions to aid internal functioning and *vice versa.*

Points can be selected from the meridian involved, its paired internal/external meridian, or its paired hand or foot six channel meridian. One may also select *a shi*, *kori,* or trigger points in the affected zones.

Acupuncture Energetics: The Broad View

A decade ago, I was at a loss to teach French meridian acupuncture since none of the source material was available in English. The available translations of Chinese language texts made little or no reference to the secondary or eight extraordinary vessels. As I taught early classes from my own translations of de Morant, Chamfrault, Van Nghi, and Schatz, I began to realize that some of the French descriptions of meridian energetics are overintellectualized and are, it seems to me, interpretive translations. This does not make them wrong, but neither does it guarantee that they are rigHt Since none of what I was teaching regarding the so-called secondary vessels was in English, I started assessing these French teachings against my own clinical experience. In that process, I began to feel that the French descriptions of these secondary vessels and especially Van Nghi's were too exact and did not correspond to my clinical experience. I was searching for a broader, more general picture or set of images of the meridian system to teach my students and share with my patients.

For me, the beginning of a solution to this problem came when a colleague took my story about acupuncture images as what we actually share with our clients quite seriously. At that time, she was just finishing her training as an art therapiSt She would have her acupuncture clients draw the disturbances they felt in their bodies. Then she would share her acupuncture images of what she felt was dysfunctional with them, asking them to draw new images of how they felt after the acupuncture sessions in the week between treatments. She put charts of all 71 meridians on the wall above her treatment table. These images not only guided her hunt for the client's problem but entered the client's descriptive vocabulary as well. Her clients found it easy to locate their problems on one or another of these acupuncture images.

Based on her experience, I came up with a written exercise for my second-year students at the Tri-State Institute of Traditional Chinese Acupuncture that I still use today. In this exercise, students pick any *zang fu* pattern they wish and reframe and reformulate this pattern in terms of acupuncture images. They check the symptoms of the *zang fu* pattern involved and search for the meridians which share these symptoms. They then chart the symptoms on pictures of the meridians. Originally, I gave no guidance on how to approach this exercise. I simply stated that the goal was to see if they could portray *zang fu* disorders in meridian terms, utilizing the *jing luo* filter instead of the *zang fu* filter.

To my surprise, almost all my students chose to draw the meridians they felt were involved on transparent acetate. In doing this, they placed one meridian image upon the next and so forth. Students would often remark that when they did this, placing several relevant acupuncture meridian images one over another, the resulting, overlapping composite image made no sense. According to my students, they were hopeless.

I, on the other hand, was elated with these images. In order to make sense of them for students, though, I started playing around with them until I was able to figure out some general patterns.

After a couple of years working with this material, I finally realized that these acetate composites amounted to entire meridian systems for particular zones. For example, if a student was portraying the meridians of the gallbladder and triple heater, from tendinomuscular to regular, as well as related extraordinary vessels running up the upper back and lateral neck in a patient suffering from rising liver fire with tinnitus and migraines, the *shao yang* zones were represented in composite fashion. In other words, all the pathways of the gallbladder and triple heater meridians, from the wider more diffuse tendinomuscular ones to the more precise longitudinal *luo* and regular meridians, as well as the extraordinary vessel, the *yang wei mai* which flows through this upper neck and head zone, were shown.

I knew from clinical experience that the majority of patients' complaints do follow these greater meridians—*tai yang, shao yang, yang ming*—but an acupuncture theory for such composite images was wanting. Then a student showed me images from a new textbook from China that showed the 12 cutaneous regions. These images also appear in Bensky and O'Connor's translation of the Shanghai College of TCM's *Acupuncture, A Comprehensive Text.* In these drawings, there are only six shaded zones even though they are referred to as the 12 cutaneous regions. Upon careful examination, I realized these were the greater meridian units depicted pictorially. This was the answer. Here, in the drawing of the cutaneous region of *shao yang*, for example, was a *broad view,* an image that included all of the pathways of *shao yang*, from tendinomuscular to divergent to *luo* to regular. This is what I had been looking for and finally everything fell into place.

The Protocol

If we take the cutaneous regions as the *surface projections of representations* of the underlying meridian pathways, as the broadest possible view of the meridian system, then, in examining and treating the cutaneous regions, one is also treating the underlying meridian systems, at least indirectly. Thus the cutaneous region of *shao yang*, for example, is a surface representation of the tendinomuscular, divergent, *luo,* and regular meridians of *shao yang*, namely the gall-bladder and triple heater. This greater meridian cutaneous region or zone is traversed by two extraordinary vessels, the *dai mai* or belt vessel, and the *yang wei mai.*

Therefore, if a patient presents with complaints and the acupuncturist's palpation also reveals constrictions throughout the area of the gallbladder and/or triple heater cutaneous region, then the *shao yang* zone which runs down the lateral aspect of the body should be the focus of the treatment. In this case, yang excess constrictions throughout the *shao yang* zone should be treated locally to release tender and trigger points, while distal points from the *shao yang* should be added to ground the treatment.

Finally, since yang tends toward excess and yin toward deficiency, while dispersing the yang excess zone of *shao yang*, we should also tonify or support the paired yin pathways, namely the *jue yin,* the liver and pericardium. While the *jue yin* may not be deficient yet, with no deficiency signs in the *hara* or pulse of the liver and pericardium, I believe we should treat it nonetheless based on the principle that when yang becomes excess, its paired yin will eventually become deficient. Shoring up *jue yin* while dispersing *shao yang* is, therefore, preventive therapy, just like tonifying spleen earth if liver wood is excess, since wood eventually invades earth according to five phase theory.

This same theory holds true for the *tai yang,* where *shao yin* should be tonified while *tai yang* excesses are dispersed, and for the *yang ming,* where the *tai yin* should be supported. In this protocol, the corresponding yin unit of the yang zone that is in excess is considered to be a core or root of the treatment. If there are also specific root imbalances, say a deficient lung pulse, then this can be tonified by whatever root treatment principles one prefers. In fact, one of the beauties of this protocol is that the root part of the treatment may be done as suggested here or by whatever root treatment means one is fond of using. What is key, however, is to focus on dispersing and releasing the yang excesses—*a shi, kori,* trigger points—in the yang zone in question.

According to this methodology, I expect recurrent and chronic pain and other holding patterns, such as constrictions, loss of range of motion, muscular weakness, and skin conditions, to occur along one of the three yang cutaneous regions—*tai yang, shao yang,* or *yang ming.* These three yang regions constitute the three major aspects of the body: the dorsal aspect, the lateral aspect, and the ventral aspect. Therefore, I have labeled these zones accordingly. There is the dorsal, *tai yang* zone; the lateral, *shao yang* zone; and the ventral, *yang ming* zone.

In evaluating a recurrent or chronic pain problem according to this system, one merely maps the complaints, as well as findings regarding tender points, onto whichever of the three zones are affected. Treatment then begins by focusing on the zone with the preponderance of symptoms and tender points, especially if it is the zone (as is almost always the case) where the patient experiences pain and related dysfunction. Points are selected from the zone in question, and distal points are selected from tender or reactive points on the same meridians. In addition, yin-tonifying points from the yin paired zone are also needled. Local and distal points from the extraordinary vessels that crisscross the yang zone in question are also treated where appropriate.

At any appropriate time, one can simplify treatment to a pure tendinomuscular, divergent, or *luo* treatment or simply treat the extraordinary vessels involved to reduce the number of needles and focus the treatment. However, for the first few treatments, I find it useful to treat an entire yang zone. One can usually pinpoint the most troubled area within a few treatments as it becomes more resistant to release by such a general approach. This can then be focused on directly.

I generally advocate treating only once a week in recurrent or chronic pain patients, although they may well wish to continue or begin some sort of physical therapy at the same time. Physical therapy should not occur on the same day as acupuncture treatment. Ideally, it should take place the day before to ready the zone for release, the day after to continue the release, or both. One can, nevertheless, be quite flexible here. I have found that weekly treatments should continue for four to six sessions, followed by a month-long break. The patient may continue physical therapy but should not begin any new form of therapy during this hiatus.

The patient should then be seen for a single treatment one month after the first series is completed with follow-ups once a month in recalcitrant cases or on an as-needed basis. It is also advisable to follow-up with a single treatment at least once every three months in chronic pain cases. This continues the release of disturbed zones, uncovers new constrictions that may arise, and accustoms the individual to pain management as an ongoing process that requires his or her compliance and active involvement.

In adopting this protocol, one makes repeated use of certain sets of points from each of the three yang zones, especially distal points, because they are so clearly effective in opening up and releasing the zones in question. Local points also come to be treated in recognizable patterns. The practitioner who palpates painful areas and feels for tender points will gain a clinical awareness of recurrent patterns of points for common myofascial pain disorders which will prove very effective. While some root treatment practitioners might criticize this as predetermined, I believe the repetitive use of point combinations that have proven clinically effective in a wide range of disorders is a major characteristic of classical acupuncture. What tailors the treatment to the individual client is the attention given to local tender points. For me, it is here that we contact the client most deeply, in his or her direct experience of distress.

In the three chapters that follow, I give guidelines for relieving yang excess and supporting the related yin zone for each of the three zones—dorsal, lateral, and ventral. I begin with the acupuncture image of the zone and the acupuncture points and meridians involved. Then follows a discussion of the muscles involved, Travell's most common trigger points for that zone, and the treatment strategies I have found effective. Discussion of each zone concludes with a case history intended to clarify the use of this protocol in clinical practice.

7

The Dorsal Zone

Acupuncture Image, Acupoints, & Meridians

The dorsal zone is comprised of the cutaneous zone, and tendino-muscular, divergent, *luo,* and regular meridians of the *tai yang* or maximum yang, namely the hand *tai yang* small intestine and foot *tai yang* bladder. This zone includes the region of the upper sinuses, forehead, top of the head, and back of the body from the occipital region and nape of the neck down the spine and muscles running paraspinally, through the buttocks and back of the thighs and calves to the outer edges of the feet and little toes. The arm branch flows up the outer edge of the arm starting at the little finger and crosses through the region of the scapula and the scalene muscles of the neck, passes through the cheek, and ends in front of the ear bilaterally. The extraordinary vessels traversing this zone are the *du mai,* running from the perineum up the spine, over the top of the head, and down the front of the forehead, ending under the nose, and the *yang qiao mai* which traverses the entire dorsal zone.

Circulation through the regular meridians follows a cycle starting with the lungs. The first breath of life brings cosmic qi and, therefore, air into the body. Thus the circulation of qi moves the blood as well as oxygenates it. This cycle ends with the liver, which controls the diaphragm. The diaphragm is essential to the lungs' respiratory function. This cycle follows through three energetic units and

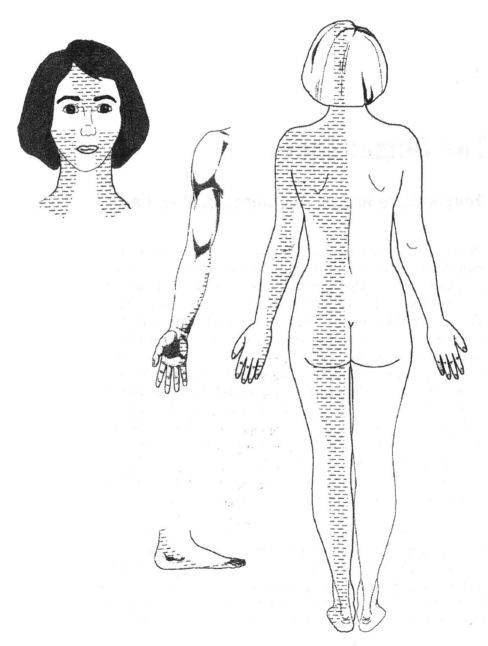

Dorsal Zone Acupuncture Image

the focus of these three units is what characterizes French meridian acupuncture.

These three units of qi circulation are: *tai yin/yang ming* (lungs, large intestine, stomach, spleen); *shao yin/tai yang* (heart, small intestine, bladder, kidneys); and *jue yin/shao yang* (pericardium, triple heater, gallbladder, liver). If we look at this cycle from a five phase perspective, it flows essentially against the generation cycle of the internal *zang fu* organs and bowels from metal to earth (*tai yin*) to fire to water (*shao yin*), back to fire, and then to wood (*jue yin*).

This order seems confusing until one looks at the cycle of meridian circulation from the perspective of the eight extraordinary vessels. These eight vessels are formed prenatally, before the first breath of life that starts the regular meridians flowing from lungs to liver as above. Therefore, some French authors refer to these as the genetic coders. They are likened to the RNA/DNA in that they code the zones of the body and lay down the energetic templates for development of the organs and bowels. According to this view, the eight extraordinary vessels are formed embryologically.

From this point of view, the *ren mai* and *chong mai,* running up the ventral aspect of the body, form the ventral zone. The *du mai* and *yang qiao mai,* running up the back of the body, form the dorsal zone. And the *yin qiao mai,* which connects with its paired *yang qiao mai,* links up the yang energies to the dorsal zone and the yin energies to the ventral zone, and the *ren mai* is where it all begins. This leaves the *yin wei mai* and *yang wei mai* connecting the upper and lower, right and left lateral zones of the developing organism, while the *dai mai,* encircling the midsection like a belt, maintains all longitudinal meridian pathways in their places.

The key points that open each of these eight extraordinary vessels in order are: Lu 7, Sp 4; SI 3, Bl 62; Ki 6; Per 6, TB 5; and GB 41. This is exactly the same order as the three units of qi circulation through the regular meridians described above, *i.e.,* metal, earth, fire, water, water, fire, and wood. Therefore, one can see that the eight extraordinary vessels prefigure the 12 regular meridians and lay down the energetic groundwork, as it were, for these 12 meridians and the 12 organs and bowels to which they are connected.

The dorsal zone itself is coded energetically by the *du mai* and *yang qiao mai*. Their reunion or opening points are SI 3 and Bl 62.

The main distal acupuncture points of the dorsal zone are: Bl 67, 64, 62, 60, 59, 58, 57, and 40; SI 3, 4, 6, 7, and 8

The main local points are:

Bl 53-54 and Bl 31-34 for the buttocks

Bl 11-25 and Bl 41-54 for the erector spinae paraspinal muscles and the *Hua Tuo jia ji* points for the multifidi lateral to the erector spinae muscles and perhaps also for the rotator muscles

Bl 10 for the occipital region

Bl 9 through Bl 3 for the occipitofrontalis muscle

Bl 1-2 for the orbicularis oculi muscle

SI 9-14 for the muscles of the scapula region

SI 16 for the scalenus muscles

SI 17 for the posterior digastric muscle

SI 18 for the zygomaticus major muscle

Distal points can, of course, be used as local points for the problems of the arms, hands, legs, and feet. In locating these points, it is necessary to begin palpation for tender points at the standard point location itself, palpating above and below the point along the path of the meridians until a constricted, tender point is identified. I believe these local reactive points are what one should needle, not the textbook locations of these points. The location of these locally constricted points often overlap with Travell's trigger points as will be seen below.

Other main dorsal zone points from the extraordinary vessels involved are:

GV 1 for the pelvic floor muscles

GV 3-4 for the low back

GV 8-9 for the mid-back

GV 13-14 for the upper back

GV 16 for the occipital region

GV 23 for the frontal sinuses and forehead

Yang qiao mai points

Bl 62 for the lower torso, legs, and feet

SI 3 for the hands and arms

SI 9 for the scapula muscles and upper back

The main meridians treated in the dorsal zone for pain management are the cutaneous region and tendinomuscular meridians of the small intestine and bladder; the divergent meridian of the bladder; and the regular meridians of the *tai yang* via their distal points; the distal points and front *mu* and back *shu* of the *shao yin* (heart and kidneys) also from the regular meridians; and the extraordinary vessel pair of the *du mai* and *yang qiao mai*.

Muscles

The following is a list by body region of the main muscles comprising the dorsal zone.

Head & neck: Middle and lower trapezius, posterior digastric, orbicularis oculi, occipitofrontalis, splenius capitus, splenius cervicus, multifidi of the neck, semispinalis cervicis, semispinalis capitis, and suboccipital muscles

Upper back, shoulder & upper arm: Levator scapulae, supraspinatus, infraspinatus, teres minor, teres major, subscapularis, and rhomboideus muscles

Torso: Serratus posterior superior, serratus posterior inferior, superficial paraspinal muscles (erector spinae muscles, namely iliocostalis thoracis, lumborum and longissimus thoracis), and deep paraspinal muscles, namely multifidi and rotatores

Lower arm & hand: Extensor carpi ulnaris, abductor digiti minimi, and flexor carpi ulnaris muscles

Lower torso: Latissimus dorsi, quadratus lumborum, pelvic floor muscles, gluteus maximus and medius, piriformis, and obturator externus muscles

Hip, thigh & knee: Hamstring muscles (biceps femoris, semitendinosus, and semimembranosus) and popliteus muscles

Leg, ankle & foot: Plantaris, soleus, gastrocnemius, tibialis posterior, flexor digitorum longus, flexor hallucis longus, abductor digiti minimi, and quadratus plantae

The interested reader should consult Travell & Simons' for details of the most common locations of the main trigger points in these muscles of the *tai yang* dorsal zone.

Trigger Points

The diagram on the next page depicts the most common trigger points in the dorsal or *tai yang* zone. The interested reader should consult Travell & Simons for specifics on these trigger points, their indications, and needling precautions.

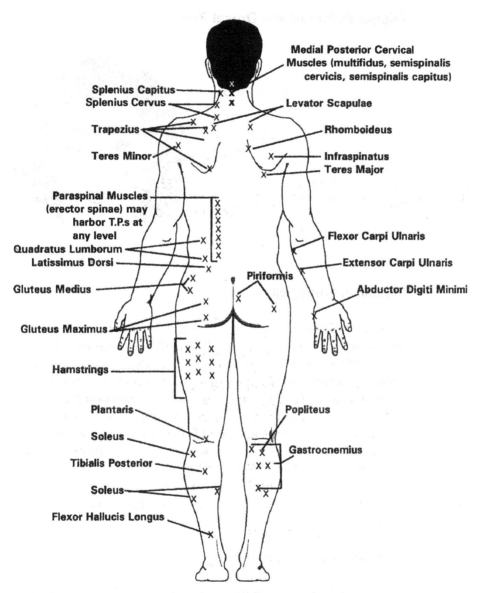

Medial Posterior Cervical Muscles (multifidus, semispinalis cervicis, semispinalis capitus)

Splenius Capitus

Splenius Cervus

Levator Scapulae

Trapezius

Rhomboideus

Teres Minor

Infraspinatus

Teres Major

Paraspinal Muscles (erector spinae) may harbor T.P.s at any level

Flexor Carpi Ulnaris

Quadratus Lumborum

Latissimus Dorsi

Extensor Carpi Ulnaris

Piriformis

Gluteus Medius

Abductor Digiti Minimi

Gluteus Maximus

Hamstrings

Plantaris

Popliteus

Soleus

Gastrocnemius

Tibialis Posterior

Soleus

Flexor Hallucis Longus

Trigger Points of the Dorsal Zone

Trigger Points of the Dorsal Zone

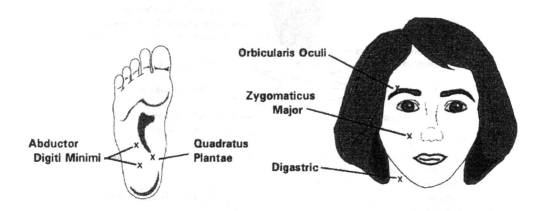

Treatment Strategies

Discussed below are common treatment strategies that I have come to rely on for myofascial pain problems of the various muscle groups of the dorsal zone. I have developed these based on a combination of Travell and Simons' trigger point therapy as described in their *Myofascial Pain & Dysfunction* and meridian-based acupuncture treatment strategies. Readers will doubtless come up with other treatment strategies or point combinations according to their own experience and style of practice. However, I believe that the key to the management of pain with acupuncture is to examine carefully for local points in the areas that trouble the patient and in all muscles connected to that area based on acupuncture and myofascial considerations.

Clearing the dorsal zone

I have found several acupuncture strategies capable of opening up the dorsal or *tai yang* zone.

1) Yang qiao mai/du mai

Because the two yang extraordinary vessels which traverse the dorsal zone serve as its energetic template, treating them is extremely effective as a first step in treating chronic myofascial pain and dysfunction in this zone. Their key points are SI 3, which opens the *du mai*, and Bl 62, which opens the *yang qiao mai*. These can be needled together to open this area and begin its myofascial release. I generally needle such points contralaterally, one on the left, one on the rigHt I select which side I treat with which point according to the patient's symptoms. For instance, if the patient suffers from pain in the muscles of the left scapula, I needle left SI 3, while needling Bl 62 on the rigHt If the patient suffers from sciatic-like pain down the back of the left hamstring muscles to the knee, I needle left Bl 62, while needling SI 3 on the rigHt One can also add local points from the *du mai* at the
level of the pain and dysfunction and/or the *Hua Tuo jia ji* points that correspond with the multifidi of the thoracolumbar spine.

I find it is wise to palpate the intervertebral and paravertebral spaces starting several vertebrae above and below the painful, dysfunctional areas. This often yields one or two exquisitely tender trigger points. These points can be needled 1/3 to 1/2 inch deep, and the needle will usually encounter significant resistance. I stop at this resistance. Holding the needle at that depth and directing it into the center of the resistance, I peck repeatedly another 1/32 of an inch or so into the dense spot, about one peck per second until the needle is grabbed. Then I leave the needle, as I do all other needles, 10-20 minutes, until the hold on the needle loosens up.

The paraspinal erector spinae muscles at the same level can be needled at the same time and in the same fashion. This usually accentuates the release. One can also needle local *yang qiao* points according to symptomatology. For instance, one can needle GB 29 for disorders of the hip, iliotibial tract, and leg or SI 10 for the upper back and scapula region.

2) Divergent meridians of *shao yin/tai yang*

The divergent meridians of the kidneys and bladder meet at Bl 40 in the popliteal crease behind the knee. Bl 10, in the occipital region on the lateral aspect of the trapezius, is also a meeting zone for the bladder and kidney divergent meridians, and the combination of Bl 10 and Bl 40 bilaterally releases spasms and stiffness of the erector spinae paraspinal muscles from the occipital to the sacral region.

In patients with paraspinal dysfunction and stiffness, I generally use this combination to open this area. I also use the combination of Bl 10 and 40 in patients with acute pain and spasm who cannot tolerate the insertion of needles directly into the affected area. I leave these needles for 15-20 minutes, thus releasing the area somewhat. I then add local tender or trigger points to effectuate a more complete myofascial release after the spasm has diminished.

3) Bl 2

Experimenting with part of a treatment strategy that Kiiko Matsumoto taught our students, I have found that needling Bl 2 where tender, anywhere from its orthodox location medial to the eyebrow to the mid-point of the eyebrow, can also release the entire paraspinal muscle network similar to Bl 10 and Bl 40.

The practitioner's hands must pinch up the flesh with the index finger on one side and thumb on the other side of the patient's eyebrow, trapping the tender spot between the fingers. I then use a very fine, 38 or 40 gauge needle with insertion tube and direct the needle swiftly 1/2 inch into the tight spot between the fingers. The skin overlying the needle often becomes quite red, and the needles should be left until this redness is greatly diminished. This takes about 20-25 minutes in most cases. It is an excellent point for patients who do not tolerate many needles, especially when in acute pain or when the paraspinal dysfunction is associated with frontal headaches. However, it should be combined with strong distal points, such as Bl 58 or 59, needled where tender or knotted.

4) Bl 14-43 plus Bl 23

As discussed in *Acupuncture Imagining*, Chapter 6, on common
stress reaction patterns in the muscles and fascia associated with
diaphragmatic constriction, I often find constriction of the rhomboid
and paraspinal muscles at the level of T5 or T6 (usually on the left)
and the iliocostalis lumborum and paraspinal muscles at the level of
L2, L3 (usually on the right). This sort of crossed, upper/lower pattern is common in chronic pain patients where repetitive wear and
tear on a particular muscle group results in what Gunn refers to as
an "injury pool." This is defined as "An accumulation of repeated
major and minor injuries to a segment leading to unresolved clinical
residuals which may, or may not, produce pain."[1]

I believe this combination is related to high stress states where the
fight-or-flight response is prolonged. This creates a chronic alarm
state. Upon questioning, these patients often report a major trauma
where they were not physically harmed but panic ensued, either at
the time of the trauma or even much later. Frequently this panic is
present continually and can be provoked by the slightest startling
event. One such startling event for these patients is simple palpation
of the paraspinal muscles in the thoracolumbar spine. The combination of Bl 14-43, needled where tight and tender, and the area
around Bl 23, also needled where most tender, is most useful in
such patients as well as in treating anxiety in general.

The image I use with such patients is of their adrenal glands stuck
in overdrive. This, I believe, corresponds to fire of the kidneys in
excess. This leads to adrenal fatigue or kidney yang deficiency
over time. In such situations, high stress patients will often report
that they are unusually energetic, real power houses, and prefer to

_____

1   Gunn, C. Chan, *Treating Myofascial Pain,* Health Sciences Center for
Educational Resources, University of Washington, Seattle, WA, 1985, p. 9

be always on the go. This corresponds to what is known as type A behavior. But they also report that they suffer from periods of severe fatigue and collapse at the end of the day. Such patients are like cars running on empty, and this point combination often produces profound relaxation. Some patients even report that they have needed to go home and rest for several hours after the first two such treatments.

Combined with distal points for the associated pericardium, namely Per 6 or 4, and the kidneys, namely Ki 2 and 3, this is an excellent relaxation treatment for patients suffering from such chronic adrenal exhaustion with its anxiety, fatigue, and panic disorders. This combination can be added very effectively to other protocols while treating these patients for myofascial pain and dysfunction in the dorsal zone.

5) Paraspinal tender points from Bl 10-32

Patients with disorders of the dorsal zone suffering from signs of a functional disorder of the nervous system may have locally tight, tender points in the paraspinal muscles at the level of the segment in which the pain is located. Gunn goes so far as to postulate that most musculoskeletal pain syndromes point to a functional dysfunction of the nervous system, classifying these as neuropathies. In such cases, Gunn states, there will be signs of sensorimotor and autonomic disturbance in the peripheral nerves. These indicate radiculopathy, whether diagnosable or not. Gunn believes that spondylosis, which is near universal and progresses with age, is the most common cause of these chronic pain syndromes. The gradual structural disintegration and changes in morphology that occur in the intervertebral discs can lead to radiculopathy.

Often this sort of neuropathy can be identified only by physical examination, since no detectable structural change may yet be present. The neuropathic nerves involved, however, discharge in an overly active, excited fashion. Such supersensitive nerves and the structures they innervate react abnormally to stimuli. This super-sensitivity of the nervous system can extend to include skeletal and smooth muscle, sympathetic ganglia, spinal neurons, the adrenal glands, sweat glands, and even brain cells. Such denervated struc-tures "overreact to a wide variety of chemical and physical inputs including stretch and pressure."[2] One of the most easily overexcited structures, Gunn continues, is striated muscle. This then leads to pain, tenderness, and increased muscle tone or spasm resulting in shortened muscles. Shortened muscles, as Travell and Simons also never cease emphasizing, exert a relentless pull that creates tugs in the myofascial fabric of the body, leading to a multitude of chronic and recurrent pain syndromes.

No pain exists in such disorders unless there is spasm. I believe this is what the classical Chinese acupuncture texts are referring to when they state that, where there is pain there is lack of free flow and where there is free flow there is no pain. The goal of treatment in such disorders is to ease this constriction and its attendant lack of free flow by removing any irritants that can be identified and by releasing the shortened muscles and the associated tender, painful spots or trigger points. Gunn stresses palpating for ropey bands of muscle shortening or, in other words, trigger points throughout the muscles in the area involved, depending on the pattern of the neu-ropathy. When there is also radiculopathy, such bands can be felt in the associated paraspinal muscles of the segment involved, and, Gunn concludes, these paraspinal bands must be released as well in such instances.

My experience with acupuncture leads me to agree. Whether one can postulate such a high prevalence of neuropathy and spondylosis as the cause of chronic musculoskeletal and myofascial pain syn-dromes or not, release of tight, shortened paraspinal muscles is very effective in such disorders. Gunn, for example, releases the trigger

_____

2   *Ibid.,* p. 8-14

points and shortened muscles of the forearm in carpal tunnel syndrome of the wriSt He also treats tight cervical muscles alongside the cervical vertebra in tennis elbow.

The dorsal zone paraspinal points of the bladder meridian can, therefore, be treated in a similar fashion, and not just for the internal medical disorders of the viscera. This is in contradistinction to TCM acupuncture where Bl 14 is used for cough, angina pectoris, chest distress, nausea and vomiting, but where no indications regarding back pain in the area of the rhomboids is even mentioned.[3]

6) Tender points, *a shi, kori,* or trigger points

Finally, one can treat any tender trigger points for myofascial pain disorders in any of the muscles of the dorsal zone. Here, one merely needs to keep Travell and Simons' texts at hand. A careful review of these texts almost always yields a very clear clinical picture of which muscles to treat. This can be accompanied by self-help home treatments and simple exercises that can be copied for the patient. Combined with supervision by a good physiatrist or other physician specializing in chronic pain and the physical therapy this physician will doubtless initiate, tender point acupuncture can be of great use and lead to much relief in:

- tension headaches affecting the occipitofrontalis muscles

- stiffness and pain in the neck due to constriction of the levator scapulae, trapezius, scalenes, posterior cervical muscles, and upper paraspinal muscles

- upper back dysfunction and pain due to constriction in thesupraspinatus and infraspinatus, rhomboids, teres major and minor, trapezius, and thoracic paraspinal muscles

---

[3]   Note that the back *shu* points for the *zang fu* can be needled for visceral disturbance along with any dorsal zone treatment for chronic pain.

- low back pain and dysfunction due to constriction of the lumbar paraspinal muscles, quadratus lumborum, and lower attachment of the latissimus dorsi

- pain, dysfunction, and sciatica emanating from the buttocks due to constriction of the gluteus medius and maximus and piriformis (including piriformis syndrome, which yields rapidly to tender point needling)

- pain and dysfunction in the hamstrings, posterior knee pain and weakness, and similar sensations in posterior sciatica

- pain and dysfunction of the calf, Achilles tendon, and heel due to constriction of the popliteus, soleus, tibialis posterior, astrocnemius, and flexor hallucis longus

- foot pain in the bottom of the foot due to constrictions in the quadratus plantae

- pain and dysfunction along the outer underside of the foot due to constriction of the abductor digiti minimi

- pain and dysfunction in the cheek due to trigger points in the zygomaticus major

- pain in the eye and headache referring to the eyebrow due to constriction of the orbicularis oculi

- upper frontal neck pain, often found in singers, due to a trigger point in the digastric muscle

- pain and weakness along the outer edge of the arm and hand due to trigger points and constrictions in the flexor carpi ulnaris, extensor carpi ulnaris, and abductor digiti minimi

The treatment of any tender points found in the above muscle groups associated with any of the above problems can be combined with other dorsal yang clearing treatments and should always be combined with strong stimulation to needles inserted into the most constricted spots near:

Bl 58-59, for pain and dysfunction of the paraspinal muscles from the occiput down to the sacrum

SI 4, 6, or 7, where tender and constricted, for disorders of the hand, arm, and scapula region

Supporting Lesser Yin

According to my protocol, one should always support the yin pair to the yang zone being released. The yin pair to *tai yang* is *shao yin* or the heart and kidney meridians. To support the *shao yin,* I prefer the *Nei Jing* use of *ying* and *shu* distal points for disorders of the yin. This means needling Ki 2 and 3. One can use instead the tonification point of the kidneys, Ki 7, if the kidney pulse is deficient or the source point alone, Ki 3, to support the kidneys. In fact, one can use any strategies one prefers to support the *shao yin* here. However, the reader should note that I follow the Japanese custom and avoid needling the heart meridian. Hence I support only the kidneys when using distal points to support the *shao yin*. One can also use the back *shu* points for the heart and kidneys for visceral dysfunction in these areas, namely Bl 15 and Bl 23. Another good combination to support the *shao yin* in a root fashion are the root and node points of the *shao yin,* Ki 1 and CV 23.

Clinical Hints

In treating the dorsal zone, it is of utmost importance that the patient be absolutely comfortable. Most pain patients cannot comfortably lie face down on a flat table with their head turned to one side and remain there for 10-20 minutes. Therefore, the practitioner should either use a table with a face hole, as well as pillows to support the abdomen and straighten the lumbar curve, or they should treat the patient lying on their side. One can also purchase table pads with head and face attachments. Personally, I prefer these.

A Case in Point

During the initial intake and physical examination, if a patient complains, for example, of frequent tension headaches starting in the occipital region but referring to the forehead, possible sinus headaches centered in the eyebrows, and a history of recurrent or chronic pain in the paraspinal muscles, buttocks, or posterior aspect of the thighs or calves, I quickly suspect that the dorsal zone is the primary area of dysfunction. The physical examination in such cases will usually yield several specific tender spots and trigger points in the flexor hallucis longus (Bl 59 area), gastrocnemius or lateral soleus (Bl 58 area), or in the plantaris muscle (Bl 40 area), especially if the problem involves recurrent or chronic myofascial pain and dysfunction in the lumbar paraspinal muscles and/or piriformis, gluteus maximus, or gluteus medius. In such cases, the quadratus lumborum muscle is often severely constricted with trigger points in the area of Bl 52-54.

According to Kiiko Matsumoto, constriction in the quadratus lumborum is related to the adrenals, and my experience certainly corroborates this. As Gunn points out, the same sort of supersensitivity that can occur in dysfunctional striated and smooth muscle can also arise in the sympathetic ganglia and adrenal glands. Patients with dorsal zone recurrent or chronic dysfunction often resemble type A individuals who feel like they are always "under the gun" and "running against the clock." Might it be that these very apt expressions characterizing such individuals are, in fact, indications that the patient has internalized these images and the sensations and the physiological stress response or sympathetic nervous system up-regulation that goes with them? Might it be that they do, in fact, suffer from "supersensitive," overly agitated, excited and excitable adrenal glands and that the surface manifestation of this adrenal irritation is the perpetuation of somatic trigger points in the quadratus lumborum and iliocostalis at the same level? In other words, quadratus lumborum constriction may be a viscerosomatic effect stemming from irritated and supersensitive adrenal functioning due to elevation of the stress response.

Palpation of the quadratus lumborum area in such individuals often elicits a severe jump sign and one indication of successful treatment is when the practitioner can finally go right to this area with the patient lying face down and palpate it directly with no jump sign. When this is achieved, such patients will spontaneously report a greater feeling of calm. They may mention that everyone has pointed out how much less stressed and anxious they are, and report that they do not collapse at the end of the day. Such patients benefit greatly from a few treatments to release the quadratus lumborum, with local trigger points as well as local Bl 22-24 where most tender. These local points will be found especially on the right, though I usually treat them bilaterally. I then combine these with strong distal stimulation at tender spots near Bl 58-59 and Ki 2 and 3 to support the *shao yin* zone. These are distal points for the Bl 23 area and have the effect of calming the adrenals.

Once the quadratus lumborum is less reactive, I spend a treatment or two releasing constrictions the length of the paraspinal muscles, needling Bl 10 and 40 to relax these muscles and adding local trigger points as indicated by physical examination. If the multifidi are constricted at any specific level, I needle these as well and add in the extraordinary vessel opening treatment for the *du mai*, SI 3 coupled with Bl 62. Distal and local treatment of the foot *shao yin* or kidney meridian is included each session. In addition, in at least one follow-up session some months later, I usually treat the root and node points of the *shao yin*, namely Ki 1 and CV 23. I often combine these with a *yin qiao mai* strategy for general relaxation that is very effective for anxious and panic prone individuals, Ki 6 and Ki 27.

If, during a follow-up visit, such a patient presents with sciatica in the lateral hip and posterior calf, with pain and restricted motion in the scapular region (infraspinatus and teres minor), stiffness of the neck and constriction in the levator scapula, and constriction in the facial zygomaticus major muscle, this is a clear indication of *yang qiao mai* involvement. The key *yang qiao mai* tender points along with Bl 62 and its coupled SI 3 are thus indicated, rather than a more generalized *tai yang* dorsal zone release.

If a specific localized acute pain syndrome develops in this zone, for instance in the upper left infraspinatus and levator scapulae following exposure to a cold draft from an air conditioner, Van Nghi's tendinomuscular protocol does suffice. This consists of needling SI 1 and TB 1, the *jing* well points, and SI 3 and TB 3. These are the tonification points for the regular meridians believed, in this case, to be relatively deficient compared to the local, excess yang meridian. One should also search for and treat tender local points near SI 11, SI 13-14, TB 15, and perhaps TB 16.

The above treatment guidelines and suggestions are presented not to limit treatment possibilities but rather to suggest a broad base from which practitioners may pick and choose those strategies they prefer and that fit the clinical case at hand. If, for example, a student of mine prefers to open the *tai yang* zone in a case such as the one above by using a specific point combination learned from Kiiko Matsumoto employing distal points outside the dorsal zone itself, I merely ask if the dorsal zone has been released by this point combination. If it has, then this to me is an acceptable treatment protocol for the dorsal zone in that case. However, the defining characteristic and *sine qua non* of this style of meridian-based acupuncture is the release of palpable myofascial constrictions.

8

Lateral Zone

Acupuncture Image, Acupoints, & Meridians

The lateral zone is comprised of the cutaneous zone, and tendino-muscular, divergent, *luo,* and regular meridians of the *shao yang* or lesser yang, *i.e.*, the hand *shao yang* triple heater and foot *shao yang* gallbladder meridians. This zone includes the temporal region and side of the head, the upper trapezius, the upper back and latissimus dorsi, the side of the hip and the iliotibial tract running along the outside of the leg, and the outside of the lower leg to the dorsum of the foot to the fourth toe. The arm branch flows up the dorsum of the forearm starting at the fourth finger. It continues up the lateral aspect of the upper arm and shoulder, along the upper trapezius and temporalis muscles and ends at the outer edge of the eyebrow. The extraordinary vessels traversing this zone are the *dai mai* encircling the waist and the *yang wei mai* which traverses the entire lateral zone.

Regarding the energetic coding of the eight extraordinary vessels, the *dai mai* serves to keep the meridians flowing and communicating longitudinally and controls rotation of the body. The *yang wei mai* serves to energize the lateral zone and connect the upper right with the lower left and *vice versa*. Thus the lateral zone is coded energetically by the *dai mai* and *yang wei mai*. The reunion or opening points of these two extraordinary vessels are GB 41 and TB 5.

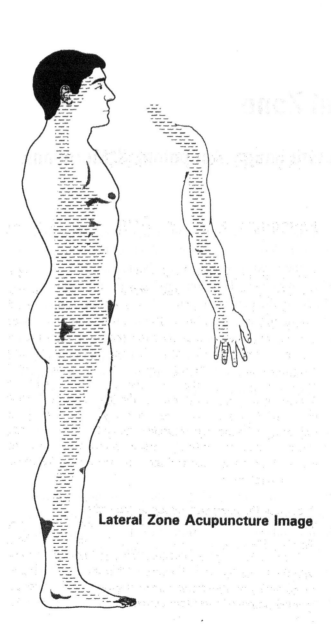

Lateral Zone Acupuncture Image

The main distal acupuncture points of the lateral zone are:

GB 44, 41, 40, 39, 38, and 34

TB 3, 4, 5, 8, and 10

The main local points are:

GB 31 for the iliotibial tract

GB 29 for the tensor fasciae latae

GB 24, 27, and 28 for the external oblique

GB 26 for the internal oblique

GB 22 for the serratus anterior

GB 21 and 20 for the upper trapezius

GB 19 and 14 for the occipitofrontalis muscle

GB 8, 6, 5, 4, and 3 for the temporalis muscle

GB 1 for the orbicularis oculi muscle

TB 9 for the finger extensor muscle

TB 14 for the supraspinatus tendon

TB 15 for the supraspinatus muscle

GB 16 for the upper sternocleidomastoid and scalenus medius muscles

TB 20, 21, and 22 for the temporalis muscle

TB 23 for the orbicularis oculi muscle

All distal points can also become local points for dysfunction and pain in the arms and hands, feet and legs. These local reactive points usually correspond to Travell's trigger points, and one should refer to her texts for guidance when needling these local points.

The main lateral zone points from the extraordinary vessels involved are:

> *Dai mai* points GB 41, 26, 27, and 28 for the external and internal obliques.

Secondarily, one may perhaps also include the iliopsoas and, therefore, Sp 10 and Liv 9 where tender for the vastus medialis and sartorius involvement in psoas pain and dysfunction and the local psoas trigger point just lateral to the rectus abdominous muscle at the level of St 27 and 28. See Travell & Simons, *Vol. II,* p. 100 for palpation of this point. While it cannot be injected directly, it can be needled over the psoas. In this case, 1/2-3/4 inch insertion with slow pecking in the direction indicated by Travell and Simons for palpation of the trigger point will often yield dramatic release of the iliopsoas. This is typically reported quite clearly and graphically by the patient as an internal muscle spasming and releasing.

The main meridians treated in the lateral zone for pain management are the cutaneous and tendinomuscular meridians of the triple heater and gallbladder; the divergent meridians of the heart and small intestine, which meet at GB 22 for the serratus anterior; the regular meridians of the *shao yang* for distal points; the distal points and front *mu* and back *shu* of the *jue yin* (pericardium and liver) form the regular meridians; and the extraordinary vessel pair, the *dai mai* and *yang wei mai.*

Muscles

The following is a list by body region of the main muscles comprising the lateral zone. Details of the most common locations of main trigger points are provided in Travell and Simons' texts.

Head & neck: Upper trapezius, temporalis, suboccipital, occipitofrontalis, orbicularis oculi, sternocleidomastoid (SCM), and scalenus medius muscles

Upper back, shoulder & upper arm: Supraspinatus, latissimus dorsi, posterior deltoid, and triceps brachii muscles

Torso: Serratus anterior, external oblique, internal oblique, and latissimus dorsi muscles

Lower arm & hand: Extensor digitorum, extensor indicis, middle and ring finger extensors muscles, and the fourth dorsal interosseus muscles

Lower torso: Gluteus medius and gluteus minimus muscles

Hip, thigh & knee: Tensor fascia latae, vastus lateralis muscles, and the collateral ligament

Leg, ankle & foot: Peroneus longus, peroneus brevis, peroneus tertius, extensor digitorum longus, extensor digitorum brevis, and the 4th dorsal and plantar interosseus muscles

Trigger Points

The diagram on the next page shows the most common trigger points in the lateral *shao yang* zone. The reader should consult Travell and Simons for specifics.

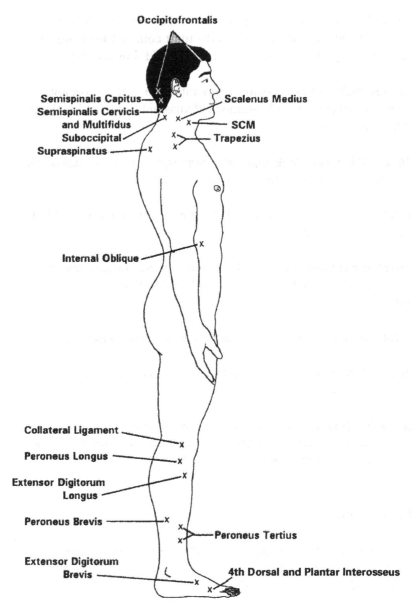

Occipitofrontalis

Semispinalis Capitus

Semispinalis Cervicis
and Multifidus

Scalenus Medius

SCM

Suboccipital

Trapezius

Supraspinatus

Internal Oblique

Collateral Ligament

Peroneus Longus

Extensor Digitorum
Longus

Peroneus Brevis

Peroneus Tertius

Extensor Digitorum
Brevis

4th Dorsal and Plantar Interosseus

Trigger Points of the Lateral Zone

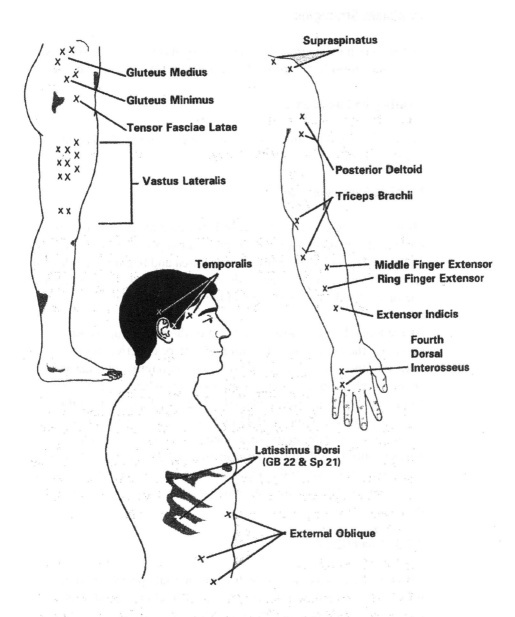

Trigger Points of the Lateral Zone

Treatment Strategies

Common treatment strategies I use for myofascial pain problems of
the various muscle groups of the lateral zone are discussed below.

Clearing the lateral zone

There are several treatment strategies for opening up the lateral zone
of the *shao yang*.

1) *Dai mai/yang wei mai*

These two yang extraordinary vessels traverse the lateral zone and
serve as its energetic template. Their reunion points, GB 41 and TB
5, can be needled together to open this area and begin its myofascial
release. Again, I usually needle these opening points contralaterally,
one on each side, chosen based on the location of symptoms.

As mentioned in the above discussion of the main acupuncture
points for the lateral zone, the *dai mai* is very effective in the
release of the lower external oblique and the internal oblique and as
an aid in releasing the iliopsoas muscle. This is accomplished by
adding the local *dai mai* points, GB 26, 27, and 28. This combination of opening points, GB 41 and TB 5, is useful for whiplash
syndrome, especially in the first stage of treatment, and helps
release contralateral, upper/lower myofascial dysfunction of torsion.
These typically involve the upper left levator scapulae and multifidi,
lower right gluteus medius and minimus, latissimus dorsi, and so
on.

2) TB 16 and GB 22

TB 16 is the union point of the triple heater and pericardium divergent meridians and is very effective for stiffness and pain in the
upper neck involving constriction of the upper sternocleido mastoid

and scalenus medius muscles when combined with TB 1 and Per 1 and local tender points.

GB 22, the union point for the divergent meridians of the small intestine and heart, is often a tender point in the lateral zone for the relief of chest pain and constriction. It is best combined with CV 17 for the area of the chest and with the root and node of the *jue yin*, Liv 1 and CV 18, for relief of constrained qi of the cheSt This may or may not be combined with the *jue yin* points, Liv 3 and 5 and Per 6 and 4.

3) GB 1 and TB 23; GB 3 and TB 22

These points are a very effective local combination for temporal headache, migraine headache, and temporal symptoms associated with TMJ. These points open up the region and prepare it for tender point needling. GB 3 and TB 22 should be needled where tender and constricted as opposed to their textbook location.

4) GB 31

Needled where tender and constricted, this point opens up the ili-otibial band and vastus lateralus muscles and readies them for tender point release.

5) GB 34

Needled where tender and constricted, this point opens up the per-oneus longus, brevis and tertius muscles and readies them for tender point release.

6) Tender points, *a shi, kori,* or trigger points

Any tender trigger point may be treated for myofascial pain disorders in any muscles of the lateral zone. Here again, Travell and Simons' texts should be kept ready for reference and prove extremely valuable for clarification of trigger points and muscles involved, for organizing treatment goals, for patient education and self-help, and for referral to physical medicine specialists if needed. In my experience, chronic pain is best treated when the acupuncturist needling tender points works in collaboration with a physician specializing in physical medicine and pain management. This may include a physiatrist, orthopedist, osteopath, or neurologiSt These typically will initiate the appropriate exercise and physical therapy regimen, of which acupuncture is an integral part. In this multidisciplinary fashion, tender point acupuncture can be very effective in the treatment of:

- tension headache and migraine headache involving constriction of the temporalis and occipitofrontalis muscles (GB 8, 6, 5, 4, and 3 and TB 20, 21, and 22 for the temporalis muscle; GB 19 and 14 for the occipitofrontalis muscle; and GB 20 and 21 and the extra point *An Mian* for the upper trapezius and suboccipital muscles)

- tension and constriction in the upper neck, especially in the case of radiculopathy, which can be aided by needling trigger points of the sternocleidomastoid and scalenus medius muscles

- upper back, shoulder, and arm pain and dysfunction due to constricted muscles and trigger points in the supraspinatus, latissimus dorsi, posterior deltoid, and triceps brachii

- pain and dysfunction under the axilla due to serratus anterior trigger points

- pain and dysfunction in the lateral aspect of the upper and lower abdomen due to myofascial constrictions in the external and internal oblique and iliopsoas

- arm and hand pain and dysfunction due to constriction of the extensor digitorum, extensor indicis, and middle and ring finger extensors

- lateral hip pain and pain down the lateral aspect of the leg (iliotibial band syndrome and sciatica) due to constriction of the tensor fascia latae, iliotibial tract, and vastus lateralis with trigger points in the area of GB 29, 31, 32, and 34

- dysfunction and pain of the collateral ligament (GB 33 needled with GB 34 and 32 below and above the ligament)

- pain and dysfunction of the lateral aspect of the leg due to myofascial constriction in the peroneus longus, brevis, and tertius (GB 34, 37, 38, and 39 needled with GB 41 and Liv 3)

- pain and dysfunction of the ankle and foot due to constriction in the extensor digitorum longus and brevis and 4th dorsal and plantar interosseus muscles

These local tender points can be combined with other opening strategies of the lateral zone and should always be accompanied by strong stimulation of needles inserted into the most constricted spots near GB 43, 41, 40, 39, 38, 37, and 34 for the leg, hip, abdominal muscles, and side of the torso; TB 4 and 5 for the wrist; and TB 3, 5, and 6 for the arm, shoulder, neck, and lateral aspect of the head and neck.

Supporting Absolute Yin

It is my strong belief that release of the *shao yang* lateral zone should be accompanied by support of its paired *jue yin*. The absolute yin or *jue yin* pair to *shao yang* is comprised of the pericardium and liver meridians. As in the case of the *shao yang*, I use specific distal protocols, for instance, Liv 2 and 3 in this case. One can also use the tonification points of the *jue yin* if their respective pulses are deficient and especially in the case of the liver. One may accomplish this with Liv 8 (supplemented by Ki 10 if one wishes, according to Shudo Denmei's liver tonification protocol and TCM theory) and Per 9. Others may prefer to use the source points instead, Liv 3 and Per 7, and any root yin support strategies are equally indicated. One can add the back *shu* and/or front *mu* points for the *jue yin*, namely Bl 14 for the pericardium and Bl 18 for the liver, either while treating the *shao yang* lateral zone with the patient on their side or after taking the lateral zone needles out. Another good generic root *jue yin* protocol is the root and node points of the *jue yin*, namely Liv 1 and CV 18.

Clinical Hints

In treating the lateral zone, one can either treat the patient face down on a body support to restore proper straightening of the lumbar curve or on the side with hips flexed and the top knee over and in front of the bottom one with a flat pillow inbetween the knees for cushioning. This lateral recumbent position facilitates stretching the latissimus dorsi and also renders all necessary lateral zone points as well as their paired yin support points on the opposite leg accessible. Using this position, however, one does have to shift the patient to the other side if the problem involves both sides. I, therefore, treat face down when both sides are affected and use the lateral recumbent position if only one side is dysfunctional.

A Case in Point

The lateral zone comes immediately to mind when patients present with the sequelae of whiplash. This is a chronic pain syndrome many months or even years after the original whiplash injury. The lateral zone is traversed by the *dai mai* and the *yang wei mai*. These two extraordinary vessels are usually disturbed in any injury involving severe rotation or whipping.

In such cases, exquisitely tender trigger points are found in the upper aspect of the sternal division of the sternocleidomastoid in the area of TB 16 as well as in the upper trapezius (GB 20 and 21 and TB 15) and supraspinatus tendon (TB 14).

One such patient reported severe pain in the side of the chest, in the region of Sp 21 and higher at GB 22. After referring him to an internist in order to rule out visceral disease, I began treatment using GB 22 and Sp 21 in the latissimus dorsi. The patient's chest pain disappeared and he experienced great relief of the trapezius pain as well. In the initial treatments, I used *dai mai* (and *yang wei mai* distal opening points, GB 41, and TB 5), along with strong reactive distal points of *shao yang*, namely GB 40 and 34 and TB 3, 5, and 9 where tender. To support the *jue yin*, I initially picked Liv 2 and 3 and Per 6. However, when the patient complained of chest pain, I added the root and node, Liv 1 and CV 18. I also needled several other local tender points in a tendinomuscular fashion, namely distal points SI 1 and TB 1, SI 3 and TB 3, and local trigger points for the levator scapula (SI 14, a tender point in the multifidus lateral to C2), the sternocleidomastoid (LI 18 and SI 16 where tender), and the semispinalis cervicis and capitus (near GB 20).

The patient was also referred for regular physical therapy after the initial series of acupuncture treatments were completed. This continued for several months with great relief of the pain. I followed up with single sessions at intervals of two, then three, then four months, at which point the physical therapist, the patient, and I felt this chronic pain problem had been essentially resolved. The patient was instructed by the physical therapist to continue with certain neck and upper back stretches on a regular basis.

9

The Ventral Zone

Acupuncture Image, Acupoints, & Meridians

The ventral zone is comprised of the cutaneous zone, and tendino-muscular, divergent, *luo,* and regular meridians of the *yang ming* or sunlight yang, namely the hand *yang ming* large intestine and the foot *yang ming* stomach meridians. The yin meridians of the foot (liver, spleen, and kidneys) flow inside this zone, and these yin meridians are, therefore, protected by the yang zone which serves as their muscular armoring.

This zone includes the major muscles of the face and front and side of the neck, especially the zygomaticus major and minor, the orbicularis oculi, the sternocleidomastoid, the masseter, the platysma, and the scalenes. From there the zone extends down the dorsum of the arm to the index finger, while another branch flows down the pectoralis, sternalis, and rectus abdominus muscles. It continues down the dorsum of the leg to the second and third toes.
All four yin extraordinary vessels, the *chong mai, ren mai, yin wei mai*, and *yin qiao mai,* traverse and energize this zone.

The front of the body is considered to be yin with respect to the back which is yang. Thus it is the yin extraordinary vessels which flow through and energetically code this ventral zone. The major muscles of this zone, however, are located in the *yang ming* zone comprised of the large intestine and stomach pathways. The major trigger points of the ventral zone are, therefore, found mostly on the *yang ming* pathways.

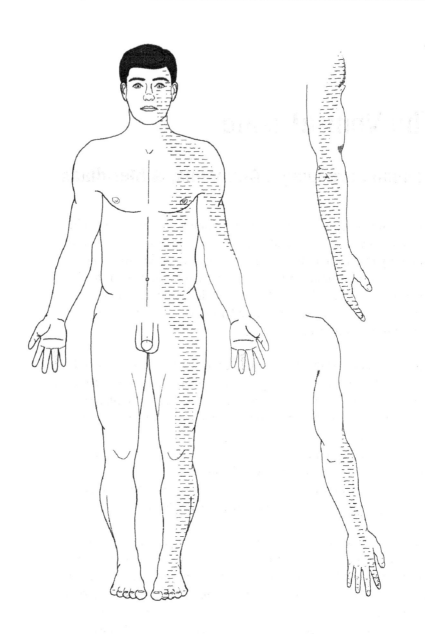

Ventral Zone Acupuncture Image

The eight extraordinary vessels are thought to operate somewhat like reservoirs of extra energy. They are called into play only if the regular channels cannot handle the work. In stress disorders of all sorts, including chronic fatigue and other immunological up-regulation conditions, the diaphragm region is often greatly restricted. This is covered in detail in Chapter 6 of *Acupuncture Imaging*. Suffice it here to say that trigger points in the *ren mai* (CV 10, 12, and 13), in the *chong mai* (Ki 11-21 and St 30), and in the pectoralis (St 13-16 and Ki 22-23) and associated areas may represent viscerosomatic effects stemming from activation of a stress response. This may refer trigger point activity to the muscles overlying the organs most disrupted by an overly activated stress response. These organs are the pericardium/heart, liver, gallbladder, large and small intestines, and pancreas.

Since these organs are irritated and rendered dysfunctional when the sympathetic nervous system remains chronically up-regulated, the regular meridians associated with them may not be able to handle the load. In this case, the job of reacting is, I believe, shifted to the extraordinary vessels and especially the *chong* and *ren*. The *chong mai* in itself often exhibits severe tender points in the rectus abdominus, sternalis, and pectoralis muscles that comprise the ventral zone over the viscera.

Thus the ventral zone is coded energetically by the four yin extraordinary vessels and especially the *chong* and *ren*. I have found that the *chong mai* reunion point, Sp 4 coupled with Per 6 for the paired *yin wei mai,* is particularly effective for opening the *yang ming* ventral zone. One can also simply use the regular meridian pair so common in TCM, St 36 and LI 4, as a distal strategy for opening the ventral zone.

The main distal acupuncture points of the ventral zone are:

St 43, 40, 39, 38, 37, and 36

LI 4, 6, 10, and 11

The main local points are:

St 36–39 for the tibialis anterior muscle

St 31 and 32 for the rectus femoris and underlying vastus medialis muscle

St 19–30 for the rectus abdominis muscle

St 18 and 16-14 for the pectoralis minor and major muscles

St 13 for the subclavius muscle (between Ki 27 and St 13, where most knotted)

St 12 for the platysma (combined with St 5 and 6)

St 9 and 10 for the sternal division of the sternocleidomastoid (most effective when combined with Ki 27 and St 13 and St 5–6 where tender to release above and below the sternocleido-mastoid, combined with the most tender and reactive trigger points in the sternocleidomastoid. See Travell & Simons for location and needling procedures, *Vol. I,* p. 202, 211-215)

St 5-7 for the masseter, and medial and lateral pterygoid muscles

St 8 for the frontalis muscle

St 3-4 for the zygomaticus major muscle

St 1-2 for the orbicularis oculi and LI 4 for the 1st dorsal interosseus muscle

LI 10 area for the brachioradialis and the extensor carpi radialis longus and brevis muscles

LI 14-15 for the deltoid and LI 15 anteriorly for the coraco-brachialis muscles

LI 13 for the biceps brachii and brachialis muscles

LI 18 for the sternocleidomastoid

LI 19-20 for the orbicularis oris

The main ventral zone points from the yin extraordinary vessels that flow through and energetically code this zone are:

St 30 and Ki 11-21 of the *chong mai* for the rectus abdominis (the most reactive trigger points usually occur at or somewhere between the kidney channel 1/2 inch from the linea alba and the stomach channel 2 inches lateral to the midline, in the center of the muscle where J. R. Worsley situates the kidney channel in his teachings.)

CV 1 of the *ren mai* for the pelvic floor muscles

CV 17-20 for the sternalis

The main meridians treated in the ventral zone for pain management are the cutaneous and tendinomuscular meridians of the large intestine and stomach; the divergent meeting zone of the *yang ming* and its paired *tai yin* at St 30; the regular meridians of the *yang ming* for powerful distal point strategies; and the extraordinary vessels of the *chong mai*, *ren mai*, *yin wei mai*, and *yin qiao mai*. One can also treat the regular and tendinomuscular meridians of the three leg yin meridians when treating the ventral zone. In pain management, the most important yin meridians are the liver and spleen regular, tendinomuscular, and cutaneous meridians. The kidney meridian of the leg is primarily treated via the *chong mai* and *yin qiao mai*.

The yin meridians of the arm, especially the lungs and pericardium, belong to no yang zone and are exceptions to the rule. Therefore, I recommend readers to consult Travell and Simons for treatment of hand and arm pain and dysfunction on the inner aspect and palmar surfaces.

Muscles

The following is a list by region of the muscles comprising the ventral zone. Travell and Simons should be consulted for details of the most common trigger points for each muscle listed.

Head & neck: Sternocleidomastoid, masseter, medial and lateral pterygoid, orbicularis oris and oculi, frontalis, platysma, and scalene muscles

Upper back, shoulder & upper arm: Supraspinatus, deltoid, cora-cobrachialis, biceps brachii, and brachialis muscles

Torso: Pectoralis major and minor, subclavius, sternalis, rectus abdominis, upper external oblique, and pyramidalis muscles

Lower arm & hand: Brachioradialis, extensor carpi radialis longus and brevis, supinator (yin associated Lu 5 area), palmaris longus (yin associated Per 5 area), hand and finger flexors (3 arm yin meridians, especially Per 6, 5, and 4 area), adductor pollicis and opponens pollicis (yin associated Lu 10 area), and the 1st dorsal interosseus muscles

Lower torso: Iliopsoas muscle

Hip, thigh & knee: Rectus femoris and vastus intermedius, and three leg yin tendinomuscular and regular meridian associated muscles—sartorius (Sp 10-Liv 9area), pectineus (Sp 12-Liv 12 area), vastus medialis (Sp 10-Liv 9 area)—and the adductor longus and brevis (Liv 10-Sp 11 area) muscles

Leg, ankle & foot: Tibialis anterior, extensor hallucis longus and brevis, 3rd and 2nd dorsal interossei, and three leg yin tendinomuscular and regular meridian associated muscles; adductor hallucis (Ki 2-4 area); flexor digitorum brevis (inferior to Ki 2), flexor hallucis brevis (Sp 3 area), adductor hallucis (Ki 1-Sp 3 area), and the 1st dorsal interosseus (Liv 3) muscles

Trigger Points

The following is a diagram of the most common trigger points in the ventral *yang ming* zone. Consult Travell and Simons for specifics.

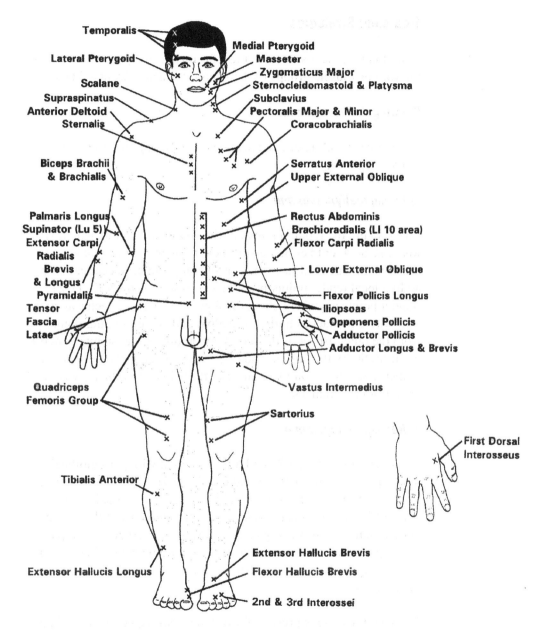

Trigger Points of the Ventral Zone

Treatment Strategies

Common treatment strategies I use for myofascial pain problems of the various muscle groups of the ventral zone are discussed below.

Clearing the ventral zone

There are several treatment strategies for opening the ventral zone or the *yang ming*.

1) *Chong mai/yin wei mai*

I have found the reunion points of the *chong mai* and its paired *yin wei mai*, Sp 4 and Per 6, are sufficient to open the *yang ming* ventral zone in a general fashion. This opening can be accentuated by adding local tender points from the *chong mai*, namely Ki 11-21 (tender points anywhere along the inner aspect of the rectus abdominus where it attaches to the linea alba) and corresponding points from the outer aspect of the rectus abdominis on the stomach meridian from St 30-19. I usually add Ki 2 and 3 to support the *shao yin* kidney, since the *chong mai* and all other yin extraordinary vessels arise from the kidneys.

2) *Ren mai/yin qiao mai*

The reunion points, Lu 7 and Ki 6, combined with periumbilical tender points (near Ki 16-15 and CV 7 and 9) and also Ki 27 effectively open the ventral zone and aid greatly in easing pain and discomfort in the umbilical region. As in all treatments of the ventral zone which overlies the organs and bowels, it is crucial that a patient's pain complaints, whether acute or chronic, be evaluated and overseen by an internist or other qualified physician to rule out visceral disease.

If visceral disease is present, for instance, colitis, peptic ulcer, hiatal hernia, or asthma, acupuncture may still prove quite helpful in alleviating the pain and discomfort. In the process of providing such pain relief, acupuncture often improves the visceral disorder, some-times even significantly. However, it is very important that such acupuncture be carried out prudently, keeping in mind the possibili-ty of the acupuncture worsening the visceral disease. The relief of pain and discomfort in visceral disease can theoretically mask important signs of aggravation, thus the need for medical collabora-tion. If, on the other hand, medical evaluation and tests prove nega-tive and visceral disease is ruled out, patients with visceral symp-toms, such as flatulence, bloating, frequent urination, chest pain, pain at McBurney's point, and dyspnea, who also complain of recur-rent or even chronic pain associated with these symptoms, may find resolution or dramatic improvement with tender point acupuncture.

3) St 36, Sp 6 and LI 4

This is a powerful combination to free up and open the ventral *yang ming* zone. When combined with St 25, a truly *yang ming* point since it is located on the stomach meridian but is the front *mu* point for the large intestine and intestinal dysfunction, CV 12, for the middle heater ruled by the *yang ming*, and Liv 3, this is a very effective strategy for opening the entire middle heater. This is because these points needled together take into account and address the liver, gallbladder, spleen, and stomach or wood invading earth.

4) CV 2-3, Liv 3, Liv 5-6, Liv 9 and Sp 8

This is an effective strategy for opening up the lower heater in cases of chronic or recurrent discomfort and associated visceral agitation in the urethra, bladder, prostate, etc.

5) *Xu Li*, St 18, CV 12, CV 17 and St 13-16

These points may be combined with distal St 43-42, St 40, and other distal reactive stomach meridian points. This is a powerful strategy for opening the upper heater, especially in the case of chest distress associated with excess heat in the upper body. This condition is evidenced by redness of the skin from the nipples on up the chest or redness of the neck and face, especially when associated with excessive heat in the stomach as in pre-ulcerous or nervous stomach patients.

6) St 30 and St 13

These points can open the entire rectus abdominis in the case of discomfort and tenderness. These can be combined to great effect with St 2 needled horizontally down the cheek and any other strongly reactive stomach meridian points.

7) Tender points, *a shi, kori,* or trigger points

One can treat any tender trigger points for myofascial pain disorders in any of the muscles of the ventral zone. Refer to Travell and Simons for details. Trigger point acupuncture can be very effective in the treatment of:

> - cluster headaches due to trigger points in the sternocleidomastoid (with St 43-42, St 40, St 39 or 37, wherever reactive; Liv 3 and LI 4 for constrained qi in general; local St 8, TB 16, GB 20 and 21 to also free up the trapezius; local sternocleidomastoid trigger points according to Travell and Simons; St 12-13 to free up the overlying platysma and attachments of the sternocleidomastoid)

> - TMJ syndrome by releasing trigger and tender points throughout the masseter and medial and lateral pterygoid (St 5, 6, and 7) as well as points to release the sternocleidomastoid and neck in general as above[1]

---

1   Kiiko Matsumoto has taught various strategies over the years at our institute for releasing the sternocleidomastoid, including Ki 6 and Ki 27; St 9, LI 18, SI 16; and St 2, GB 1, Bl 2, all of which prove very effective in such instances.

- frozen shoulder and other similar myofascial pain disorders
involving the anterior deltoid, coracobrachialis, biceps brachii,
and brachialis muscles, including thoracic outlet syndrome or
similar neck-shoulder complaints (St 13, 14, Sp 20, GB 22,
Lu 1 and 2, trigger points in these muscles, and spots that are
reactive directly behind these shoulder points for the supraspinatus—LI 16 and, SI 11-13 areas)

- chest discomfort in anxious patients (often suffering from
clinically diagnosed panic disorder) due to myofascial
constriction in the pectoralis minor and major, subclavius,
sternalis, upper external oblique and upper rectus abdominis
muscles (St 13-16; St 18, Sp 20 and Lu 1; Ki 22-27; CV 17-
18; and points to deconstrain the liver in general and the middle heater in particular if it is constricted, as it usually is in
such cases—Liv 3, Liv 5-6 where tender and reactive, LI 4,
CV 10, 12, and 13 or rectus abdominis trigger points lateral to
these areas, whichever prove most reactive, rounded out by
distal *chong mai/yin wei mai* opening points to clear the ventral zone—Sp 4 and Per 6)

- myofascial pain syndromes and repetitive strain injuries
affecting the radial dorsal aspect of the arm and inner and palmar aspects of the arms and hand (LI 1, 2, 4, 5, 6, 10, 11, 12,
14, 15, 16, 17, and 18 where tender areas coincide with trigger points in the 1st dorsal interosseus, extensor carpi radialis
longus and brevis and brachioradialis, anterior deltoid,
supraspinatus, scalene, and sternocleidomastoid muscles, all
involved in repetitive strain injuries extending down the arm
from cervical radiculopathy; following Gunn's lead, I always
add tender constricted points in the posterior cervical muscles,
i.e., multifidus, and other paracervical muscles; I add other
ventral zone points for the upper torso if constricted, and yin
palmar points if tender and involved such as Lu 5 for the
supinator, Per 5 for the palmaris longus, Per 4, 5, and 6 for the
hand and finger flexors, and trigger points near Lu 10 along
with the *jing* well point, Lu 11, for the adductor pollicis and

opponens pollicis combined with LI 4 angled toward Lu 10, LI 6, and Lu 7 angled down toward the index finger)

- myofascial pain and dysfunction of the iliopsoas. Here tender point acupuncture provides significant and often very rapid relief and resolution when combined with physical therapy stretches on a regular basis after the acupuncture treatments are concluded. The psoas is traversed by the three leg yin, liver, spleen, and kidney channels, the *chong mai*, the stomach meridian, and the *dai mai*. Therefore, acupuncture points that are reactive near St 31, St 30, Ki 11-13, Liv 9-12, and Sp 10 should be needled along with distal points Sp 8 and Liv 3, 5–6, plus Sp 4 to open the *chong mai* and the *luo* of the spleen, and St 25-27 where reactive. These may be combined with Travell and Simons' psoas trigger points (near GB 27 and Sp 12; see Travell and Simons, *Vol. II,* p. 90). When releasing the iliopsoas, I also release the three leg yin, as stated above, to release the sartorius and vastus medialis. I often round out this treatment with an "infinity treatment" I learned from Kiiko Matsumoto. This consists of treating the *chong mai* and *dai mai* which together flow through the entire iliopsoas muscle. This is accomplished by needling Sp 4 and GB 41 with their respectively paired Per 6 and TB 5. In this case, I treat contralaterally. Therefore, Sp 4 is needled on the right, Per 6 is needled on the left, GB 41 is needled on the left, and TB 5 is needled on the right

- myofascial pain and dysfunction of the quadriceps group associated with release of the iliotibial band (GB 29, 31-32 where tender) and the sartorius, vastus medialis, adductors longus and brevis and pectineus, if appropriate, using distal reactive points on the three leg yin channels to further release these muscles of the inner thigh

- myofascial pain disorders of the dorsal aspect of the leg and foot due to constriction in the muscles traversing that region, especially the tibialis anterior and extensor hallucis longus and brevis (St 36-37 for the tibialis anterior, St 39 and 41 for the extensor hallucis longus, and St 42-43, for the extensor hallucis brevis, all where reactive)

As with the other two zones discussed above, clearing surface yang excess myofascial and cutaneous constrictions should be combined with support of the corresponding yin, namely the *tai yin* or the spleen and lung meridians.

Supporting Greater Yin

The *tai yin* or greater yin comprised of the spleen and lung meridians can be supported as with the other two yin paired zones by needling the yin of yin, Sp 2 and 3. One can also use just Sp 3, the source point, or just the tonification point, Sp 2. Shudo Denmei suggests treating the most constricted reactive points anywhere from Sp 2 till just distal to Sp 4. These should be combined with Sp 6 for the three leg yin or with St 36 as a *yang ming/tai yin* regulatory strategy, plus Lu 9 and 10, just Lu 9, or Lu 7. This last point is best combined with Ki 6 to initiate a *yin qiao mai/ren mai* release of the ventral zone at the same time as supporting the core with extraordinary vessel treatment. The front *mu* and back *shu* points for the spleen and lungs can also be added. These are Liv 13 and Bl 20 for the spleen and Lu 1 and Bl 13 for the lungs. These should be added especially if there are related visceral symptoms of these organs.

Clinical Hints

As stated above, when treating myofascial pain and dysfunction of the ventral, thoraco-abdominal region, one must be very careful to insure that tender points related to visceral agitation are solely somatovisceral in nature. If the local discomfort is of a viscerosomatic origin, tender point acupuncture can still be used for relief of the somatic, cutaneous, and myofascial component *only* when medical supervision of the overall case is provided. I cannot stress this enough. In my opinion, acupuncture, from either a tender point, TCM, or Five Element perspective, is often remarkably effective for visceral distress in the organ functions of a somatovisceral and sometimes even viscerosomatic origin, but I believe good medicine requires medical supervision of the case by a physician qualified to oversee and monitor such internal medical conditions.

When treating the ventral zone face up, one should be careful to prop up the knees of patients with back pain. This back pain should also be addressed, either by treating the patient first ventrally, then dorsally, or following a series of a few ventral treatments with some to relieve the dorsal zone. This is especially true for patients suffering from mid and low back pain, where a combined release of the paraspinals and rectus abdominis is often the key to lasting relief from back pain. This is analogous to the fact that abdominal strengthening exercises are always combined with stretching and releasing the back muscles in physical therapy for such patients.

A Case in Point

The following is a case of an opera singer plagued by cervical radiculopathy, TMJ syndrome, and frequent pain and somatovisceral throat symptoms. It illustrates the effects of repetitive strain of specific muscle groups leading to visceral agitation of the internal structures underlying the myofascial zone thus irritated.

The patient presented with cervical radiculopathy, neck pain, and a history of TMJ, all of which grew more aggravated when she performed. The repetitive strain of singing seemed to be too great, and she had more or less decided to shift her focus to teaching. Her TMJ had improved significantly through the help of a dentist specializing in myofascial pain syndrome in TMJ, and regular physical therapy had helped her neck greatly, but the radiculopathy remained.

My initial examination revealed tender trigger points throughout the sternocleidomastoid, levator scapula, and scalene. More careful examination yielded trigger points in the masseter, platysma, and subclavius muscles. When pinched between the fingers, the platysma trigger points referred sensations down the arm, as did palpation of the subclavius muscle and scalenes. In this case, I combined local trigger points with a *yang ming* ventral opening protocol: LI 4, 10, 11, and 12, Liv 3, St 36, and St 12 and 13, rounded out with a *yin qiao mai* treatment at Ki 6, the paired Lu 7 for the *ren mai*, and Ki 27. After a few sessions and after major release of a specific, exquisitely tender trigger point in her right sternocleidomastoid, the radiculopathy was gone. Note that tender points near LI 17 for the scalenes and LI 18, St 9 and 10, and SI 16 for the sternocleidomastoid were needled, as were GB 20 and 21 for the trapezius, all in tendinomuscular fashion.

Release of the platysma trigger points seemed to be the key element in resolving the radiculopathy, perhaps releasing indirectly the scalenes and sternocleidomastoid muscles. This patient still comes for treatment on an as-needed basis, roughly once every 4-6 weeks, and has physical therapy far less often, once weekly or less. She has been able to resume her demanding singing career with far less pain and dysfunction. On one follow-up, she presented with throat pain, a constant with singers of course, and palpation of the sternocleidomastoid uncovered a trigger point that referred pain to the exact spot in her throat that was painful. Whether this was an instance of a somatovisceral or a viscerosomatic effect was unclear, since she was being treated both by her throat specialist for the throat irritation and by me. In any case, I have experienced great success treating singers by focusing on release of the muscles of the neck overlying the throat.

10

Acupuncture & Dry-needling

When I encountered Travell's work, I was very excited indeed, for here was confirmation of tender point acupuncture from a totally different perspective. The main drawback to Travell's trigger point injection approach seems to be the reluctance of physicians to try her technique. This is due to their lack of familarity with the location and isolation of trigger points for needling. Physician friends of mine who have read Travell and Simons' descriptions of trigger point injection, including the depth of insertion often required and the thickness of the hypodermic needle, feel that, in the wrong hands, this could be a dangerous procedure. Some colleagues of Travell and Simons have criticized the use of cortisone and Lidocaine as potentially harmful to the local tissue injected. Others have developed dry-needling as a way to get the good results of trigger point therapy without the above drawbacks. Dry-needling refers to the use of a needle alone with nothing being injected. This achieves quite good results.

C. Chan Gunn, a physician specializing in pain management who is familiar with Travell's work and with acupuncture, prefers to needle tender and trigger points with acupuncture needles. He feels these needles, which are much finer and sharper than hypodermics,

> . . . minimize trauma to the nerves and other tissues. The fine needle allows multiple, closely spaced (sometimes only a few millimeters apart) insertions into individual muscle fasciculi. The whippy nature of the fine needle transmits the char-

acter of the penetrated tissue (*e.g.*, fibrous tissue) to the therapist; the procedure is therefore also diagnostic, locating spasm
and fibrous contractures in deep muscles where they are otherwise undetectable.[1]

When I began needling Travell's trigger points as part of my local
needling protocol for pain disorders, I found that the needles often
met with significant resistance. At first I tried to push past this
resistance which is usually encountered only 1/2 inch or so deep.
But too often the thin needles I prefer to use (34-36 gauge) bent if
the muscle being needled contracted during insertion. Dr. Steven
Finando, a colleague of mine, experienced the same problem, and
we independently discovered that, if we inserted very superficially
at first, over but not into the trigger points we had fixed between the
fingers and thumbs of our left hands, and then pecked a few times
into the resistance, the patient's muscle would twitch and then grab
the needle. If the pecking was continued in a fanning fashion in several directions, lifting to the surface and then redirecting the needle
point in a new direction into the resistance, the muscle would twitch
repeatedly and then grasp the needle even more firmly.

Gunn stresses the need to obtain this needle grab or grasp which in
Chinese acupuncture is referred to as *de qi* or the arrival of the qi.
Gunn, therefore, defines dry-needling as the induction of a muscle
spasm much as do the Japanese. Finando and I have found that shallow insertion and slow penetration until resistance is met followed
by repeated gentle pecking *with no rotation or twirling of the needle*
results in far more effective needle grabs than do thevigorous lifting
and thrusting and twirling techniques of TCM acupuncture. We also
find that needling over trigger points produces the most pronounced
needle grabs as compared to needling acupuncture points by textbook location. This technique leads to muscle fasciculation as well.
Gunn states that his intramuscular technique, with the same depths
as trigger point injection, "can occasionally actuate muscle to fasci-

---

1   Gunn, C. Chan, *op. cit.*, p. 39

culation; this is usually accompanied by near-instantaneous muscle relaxation."[2]

When a fasciculation is produced, patients often report a cramp-like sensation which some describe as painful, some as strange, or indescribable. This sensation typically dulls quickly, and leaving the needles in place 10-20 minutes is usually sufficient to effectuate a release. Gunn states that insinuation of the needle into the spasm slowly, which he always does for very sensitive patients, can minimize the pain. We believe this is the method of choice for all patients not only because it is less painful but because it seems to lead the muscle more easily to fasciculate. This then results in more favorable and more rapid myofascial release. This technique also requires both far less-deep insertion and the use of much finer needles than either Gunn's intramuscular stimulation or Travell's trigger point injection or dry-needling.

When Finando and I met with Travell during her seminar at our institute, we queried her carefully about our relatively shallow needle insertion technique. We often seemed to be needling over but not actually into the trigger points themselves. She suggested that this technique is similar to spray-and-stretch and that, perhaps, we were needling into the "skin representation" of the trigger points rather than into those points directly. The experience I have had with dramatic release of the iliopsoas muscle, needling only to 1/2 to 3/4 of an inch deep with a 34 gauge needle over the proximal psoas trigger point described by Travell, has convinced me of this "skin representation" effect. The acupuncture tender point protocols I have developed, described in chapters 7-9, are based on this surface concept known as the cutaneous regions in acupuncture. Ancient Chinese texts talk about needling as a kind of fishing. *De qi* is likened to a patient casting of one's line into the water, waiting for the slightest bite. Superficial insertion followed by slow insinuation

---

2   *Ibid.*, p. 16

of the needle as described above is, I believe, like fishing and lands the desired response.

Patients should be told they may feel soreness and fatigue for a day or so after treatment. This is similar to postexercise soreness and discomfort. The application of heat to the treated areas the night after the treatment will bring some relief of this discomfort and continue the myofascial release. This can be accomplished with a hot Epsom salts bath, a shower, a hot water bottle, or a hot pack. While the muscles may feel quite sore the first day or so, many patients report that it is better within minutes or hours after treatment. When asked to explain, many describe a feeling of loosening of the constriction and improved movement. I believe this is the subjective experience of their muscles lengthening after release of the contracted muscular knots and bands. [In addition, Travell advocates stretching, either spray-and-stretch or self-stretching, after needling. For ready reference, these stretches are supplied in her two volume text coauthored with Simons.] In my experience, combining this sort of dry-needling technique with leaving the needles passively retained for 10-20 minutes produces lengthening of the constricted muscles and powerful myofascial release often not obtainable by other physical means. This passive retention phase is common to most American acupuncture treatment but has not previously been a part of dry-needling. It allows the generalized, systemic relaxation response characteristic of acupuncture to set in, thus relaxing the entire somatic ground within which local constrictions exist as especially tense or stressed areas.

I advocate using only disposable, stainless steel needles with guide tubes so that they may be inserted cleanly and effortlessly without touching the needle shaft. Clean needle technique, entailing washed hands, clean field, and sterile needles, must be followed. While it is relatively rare for acupuncture points to bleed, this is possible. This is especially possible when needling tender and trigger points that grab the needle vigorously or when needling into densely fibrotic areas. If bleeding occurs, pressure with a cotton ball or sterile gauze should be applied for a few minutes to minimize bruising or

swelling in the area. Application of a bandage over a cotton ball at
the site further minimizes bruising.

The technique I am suggesting here is very simple for any acupuncturist or medical professional trained to give injections. It is also
quite safe.

11

Acupuncture Tender Point Therapy for Acute, Recurrent, & Chronic Pain

Pain management includes the treatment of acute, recurrent, and chronic pain and their related dysfunctions. Acute pain is easily treated by tender point acupuncture, as it is by Travell's myofascial release and Gunn's intramuscular stimulation. All these approaches focus on contracted muscles harboring tight, ropey bands or, in other words, trigger points. Release of these constrictions often resolves the acute pain complaint, restores normal range of motion, and requires no follow-up or physical therapy. Acute pain disorders may be precipitated by such causes as sudden or wrenching movement, lifting a heavy object the wrong way or simply attempting to lift too heavy an object, chilling of the muscle, poor sleeping position or an unfamiliar mattress. As long as the causative event is not repeated, tender point deactivation therapies are successful and sufficient. Here tender point acupuncture offers a very effective approach that is relatively noninvasive compared with the other trigger point needle therapies described above.

Recurrent and chronic pain, on the other hand, are much more complex problems. Their treatment has become the central focus for a whole new group of pain management specialists. This includes physiatrists, orthopedists, neurologists, osteopaths, physical therapists, and, often but not always effectively, acupuncturists. Gunn and

Travell and Simons have written comprehensive Western anatomical and biological explanations for the phenomena of chronic pain. These descriptions and the therapeutic principles based on them can be applied to the acupuncture treatment of recurrent and chronic pain. Below I summarize and recapitulate these principles and procedures. As this summary, I hope, will show, acupuncture can and should be practiced according to these most current and detailed theories and principles. Acupuncture practiced from this perspective is not only extremely effective for the treatment of chronic and recurrent pain, but allows the acupuncturist to be integrated into the modern multidisciplinary management of pain. This is because all members of such a team can talk to each other using the same concepts and terminology.

Travell and Simons cover the topic of chronic myofascial pain in the conclusion to Volume II of their text. Here the authors state clearly that the chapters on individual muscles in Volumes I and II of *Myofascial Pain and Dysfunction: The Trigger Point Manual* deal essentially with myofascial pain syndromes of single muscles and their myotonic units. These acute myofascial pain disorders are usually traceable to a precise onset which is easily identified by the patient. More often than not, it is due to a temporary overload of a muscle or muscle group. It is also possible for active trigger points to become latent on their own in the absence of overload. In this case, there may be dysfunction, but there is no pain. Recurrence of a similar overload leads to reoccurrence of the pain. If the perpetuating factors are severe enough, a chronic myofascial pain syndrome may develop.

The treatment of chronic pain, that is to say pain of an enigmatic nature for which no organic cause can be found, largely remains an unresolved health care problem. It is trying and expensive for patients and frustrating for their practitioners. Most chronic pain sufferers have been told at least once that their pain is not real, that it is all in their head, that it is psychogenic in origin. Travell refers to this labelling as "the ultimate indignity."[1] Travell urges,

> Above all, *clinicians must believe that their patients hurt as much and in the way that they say they do.* The patients are describing their suffering. (Travell) discovered and mapped the referred pain patterns by believing her patients, even though they described pain in areas that were originally unexplainable.[2]

Travell stresses that most patients are *function oriented* and want "nothing more than to obtain enough understanding to control their pain so that they can return to a normal lifestyle."[3] In such patients, comprehensive trigger point treatment usually proves quite success-ful. Such comprehensive treatment involves, a) correction of any perpetuating factors, especially mechanical ones, b) management of each single muscle syndrome by releasing the trigger points present, c) stretching of the muscles through initiation of a home program of stretching and exercise, and d) education. The primary goal, Travell and Simons stress, is to teach patients how to recognize these spe-cific trigger point problems. This means to recognize and relate to these as a *gestalt*. In *Acupuncture Imaging*, I emphasize that what meridian-based acupuncturists do well is reframe or image our patients' complaints in terms of the acupuncture meridian network. This validates their experience of pain by mapping it carefully onto an image that is presented as thousands of years old but which the patients also know is correct since it corresponds to their own sub-jective experience. Similarly, Travell advocates what might be called myofascial trigger point imaging.

I believe that the protocols presented in chapters 7-9 of this book facilitate this myofascial mapping by "acupuncturizing" this pro-

---

1   Travell & Simons, *op. cit.*, Volume II, p. 542

2   *Ibid.*, p. 543

3   *Ibid.*, p. 544

cess. If I am correct, the acupuncture images called meridians are but early maps of myofascial pain and dysfunction made by acupuncturists thousands of years ago without the benefit of dissection and autopsy. Thus they lack myofascial and anatomical sophistication. Nevertheless, by locating points based on physical examination for tight, reactive, tender points that resonate with their patients' problems, the original acupuncturists were following the same procedure later adopted and advocated by Travell. In my experience, modern TCM acupuncturists often fail to take their patients' pain seriously when it is chronic and complex. Too often they trade a seemingly precise, internal, *zang fu* diagnosis for a careful physical examination of local, painful, dysfunctional areas. A tender point acupuncturist will heed Travell and the early classical acupuncturists, knowing that where there is pain, there is usually also palpable constriction. Furthermore, when this local constriction is released, the pain is typically eradicated.

However, while Travell has been brilliant in her careful mapping of myofascial pain, my experience with most practitioners of trigger point injection therapy is that they often do not map as carefully as Travell would have them. This is partly out of unwillingness to spend the time involved and partly out of a frustration with the complexity such mapping sometimes involves. In teaching physicians tender point acupuncture, I have found that the protocols described above facilitate this mapping by giving practitioners three broad zones in which to search. For example, in screening the entire dorsal zone in patients with chronic back pain, many of the single muscle patterns described by Travell will be located. Further, these will be seen to form a *functional cluster* or network that is most effectively treated by systematically releasing the entire zone as well as the focal sites of constriction and dysfunction. The acupuncture imaging protocol developed herein thus enables a practitioner to become more accurate and efficient in searching for trigger points. It also teaches the habits that lead toward developing the attitude and skill advocated by Travell.

I would stress that all patients with recurrent and chronic pain be referred to a physician specializing in chronic pain who is familiar with both Travell's trigger point therapy and the acupuncturist's tender point approach. This enables a careful examination for perpetuating factors. It also is to initiate the proper physical therapy for both in office and at home stretching. I have found a physiatrist, a medical doctor trained in physical medicine and rehabilitation, to be the best choice for such a referral. However, some neurologists, osteopaths, and orthopedists trained in myofascial work are also possible referrals. The key is that the physician be willing to hunt for any sources of pain that have been previously overlooked. Acupuncturists are, in my opinion, not sufficiently trained in Western physical medicine to conduct this screening. My 15 years' experience has shown me that, while I can often uncover areas overlooked by the patient's previous physician by carrying out the acupuncture mapping described above, diagnosis by a physiatrist can more accurately pinpoint the problem. In this case, my tender point acupuncture becomes a part of a multidisciplinary approach. In addition, chronic pain patients sometimes need antidepressants, at least for short periods of time. This is especially so if they are pain oriented as opposed to function oriented. The physiatrist or other physician specializing in chronic pain can order these medications and make further appropriate referrals. Acupuncturists should not try to play doctor by doing without this crucial screening and oversigHt

It is my belief that the physical therapy provided by acupuncturists is the work upon which we should focus. Practitioners who work in this fashion will quickly build a referral network of physicians practicing pain management. These physicians will themselves quickly become familiar with the effectiveness of this tender point acupuncture. Many acupuncturists and especially novices practicing in this way would do well to work with such specialists in chronic pain centers. The institute which I direct is dedicated to making such alliances more and more common so that tender point acupuncture may become a routine part of mainstream, multidisciplinary pain management.

Gunn, a specialist in multidisciplinary pain management, has developed a theory that much chronic musculoskeletal pain is neuropathic in origin. According to Gunn, this is, more often than not, due to an undiagnosed or "invisible" radiculopathy stemming from irritation of the nerve root. Gunn postulates that this is due to the near universal spondylosis attendant upon aging. According to this view, even when undiagnosable by current screening tests, irritation over time at the nerve root forms a pool of minor injuries that predispose a particular segment of the nervous system to dysfunction. Such dysfunction takes the form of supersensitivity and hyperirritability. Gunn believes this irritates the segment involved at the nerve root and leads to radiculopathy. In addition to advocating release of local trigger points and tight bands in the muscles, Gunn stresses the need to decompress nerve roots compressed by paraspinal shortening. Therefore, he advocates always checking for trigger points and tight bands in shortened paraspinal muscles lateral to the nerve roots of the segment involved. Dry-needle release of these paraspinal constrictions forms a key part of his program of chronic pain management.[4]

Whether or not Gunn's "neuropathy pain model" is correct, his advice to always assess and release the dorsal zone in all chronic pain patients is, in my experience, an excellent idea. In such patients, there is often significant nervous system agitation. These patients are often easily irritated muscularly. In particular, the paraspinal muscles over their adrenal glands may be especially sensitive. The acupuncture treatment of the *tai yang* and kidneys discussed in Chapter 8 is extremely effective in such cases and includes needling of these areas. Gunn stresses that patients characterized as anxious will typically be constricted in what he refers to as their "stress muscles." These are the muscles that are called into action by fight-or-flight situations. These muscles are mostly found within the dorsal zone and include the trapezius, paraspinals, infra-

---

[4]   Gunn, *op. cit.*, p. 119-20

spinatus, and gluteus maximus and medius (*tai yang*) as well as the masseter and the sternocleidomastoid (*yang qiao mai* and the ventral zone *yang ming*).

Tender point acupuncturists who always check the dorsal zone in chronic pain patients, releasing myofascial and paraspinal constrictions there, are addressing Gunn's key focus of treatment. As mentioned above, Gunn stresses relief from spondylitic radiculopathy whenever present by treating the dorsal musculature. This restores efferent flow of motor impulses and releases all involved muscle shortening. According to Gunn, the best method for accomplishing these aims is dry-needling. In essence, Gunn is stating that dry-needling is the most effective form of physical therapy for recurrent and chronic pain and dysfunction. Dry-needling stimulation "lasts longer than other forms of physical therapies, probably through the generation of a current-of-injury which can continue for days" and may also "provide a unique therapeutic benefit: it can promote healing by releasing a growth factor."[5]

The injury potentials generated by a needle when inserted into a muscle are even further prolonged in neuropathy since the area is already hyperirritable. This can be augmented by stimulation of the needle until the muscle visibly fasciculates. This fasciculation results in release of the muscle spasm and normal lengthening of the muscle. As Travell and Simons have shown, lengthened muscles do not harbor trigger points. Further, the current-of-injury released can last for days until the microwounds due to needling heal. Based on the above considerations, I suggest treatment only once per week even for chronic pain patients. This enables the body to experience the entire current-of-injury cycle that is thought to last about six days. According to this theory, microwounds, including those from acupuncture, heal in three stages, from the deepest tissue to the most superficial, over a period of just under one week.

_____

5   *Ibid.*, p. 118-20

Gunn concludes that, unlike other types of physical therapy, dry-needling stimulation not only leads to pain relief and relaxation of the muscles of a single region but

> . . . can spread to the entire segment, suggesting a reflex mechanism involving spinal modulatory systems. Sympathetic hyperactivity also responds to reflex stimulation, and the relaxation of smooth muscle can spread to the entire segment releasing vasospasm and lympho-constriction.[6]

This myofascial release and calming of the nervous system restores the tissues of the body to normalcy, thus allowing all circulatory systems, including the connective tissue network that is the "supportive network"[7] of the human organism as a whole, to flow properly.

Thus it can be seen that the complex communication carried out by the connective tissues which flow through and traverse the entire myofascial system is clearly aided in its normal functioning by myofascial release. This has long been known by trigger point therapists and bodyworkers. French acupuncturists have long felt that acupuncture, especially when it includes core energetic stimulation and release of the eight extraordinary vessels, treats the connective tissue network directly. Some Japanese acupuncturists have even called acupuncture connective tissue therapy. This network of connective tissue structures serve as the blueprint coding the rest of the bodymind's growth. It also serves as a precursor to the bones, organs, and other systems of the human organism just as the extraordinary vessels are thought to do. Perhaps this is the key to what Chamfrault and Van Nghi have referred to as "human energet-

---

[6]   *Ibid.*, p. 118

[7]   Deane, Juhan, *Job's Body: A Handbook for Bodyworkers*, Station Hill Press, Tarrytown, NY, 1987, p. 75-87

ics" in their book of the same name.[8] This is why I advocate supporting the core or root by extraordinary vessel strategies to open whichever of the three zones is the focus of treatment at the same time as supporting the paired yin zone. For instance, when the *jue yin* is needled for constriction and contraction involving the *shao yang*, this further supports the root while tender point acupuncture in the local region directly releases constrictions in the fabric of the bodymind.

Conclusion

In acupuncture imaging and tender point needling as described above, we begin by mapping a patient's chronic or recurrent pain complaints onto one of the three yang myofascial zones—dorsal, lateral, or ventral. This results in an image of the patient's holding patterns that guides tender point location and release of cutaneous and myofascial constrictions. It is my hypothesis that the acupuncture meridian system, when seen simultaneously from classical tender point and modern myofascial perspectives, is a key to understanding why individuals are *predisposed to develop recurrent and chronic myofascial constrictions, pain, and dysfunction in specific holding patterns and not in others.* It is my hope that this book will inspire American acupuncturists to return to an appreciation of classical acupuncture informed by a modern myofascial, trigger point framework. At the same time, I hope this book also inspires mainstream specialists in pain management to take a closer look at the acupuncture meridian network and the myofascial chains it describes.

Doubtless, some will say that the protocols developed herein stray from Chinese acupuncture, that they overly Westernize acupuncture or play down acupuncture in its own rigHt To these critics, let me merely reply that, for me, one of the beauties of classical and mod-

_____

8   Chamfrault, André and Van Nghi, Nguyen, *L'Energetics Humaine*, Charente Publishers, Angouleme, France, 1969

ern acupuncture is that there are a multiplicity of ways in which it can be practiced. It is my belief that this variety helps us better treat our patients and their suffering. As an American practitioner, I do not feel in any way obligated to accept any other culture's ideological beliefs about acupuncture and how it should be practiced. I feel that a new American acupuncture is currently in the making, informed by this wonderful multiplicity of approaches from many cultures. I envision this new acupuncture moving beyond old ideologies, basing its worth and its work on what helps patients in distress.

Index

OTHER BOOKS ON CHINESE MEDICINE AVAILABLE FROM:
BLUE POPPY PRESS
5441 Western, Suite 2, Boulder, CO 80301
For ordering 1-800-487-9296 PH. 303\447-8372 FAX 303\245-8362
Email: info@bluepoppy.com Website: www.bluepoppy.com

ACUPOINT POCKET REFERENCE by Bob Flaws
ISBN 0-936185-93-7
ISBN 978-0-936185-93-4

ACUPUNCTURE & IVF by Lifang Liang
ISBN 0-891845-24-1
ISBN 978-0-891845-24-6

ACUPUNCTURE FOR STROKE REHABILITATION
Three Decades of Information from China
by Hoy Ping Yee Chan, *et al.*
ISBN 1-891845-35-7
ISBN 978-1-891845-35-2

ACUPUNCTURE PHYSICAL MEDICINE: An Acupuncture
Touchpoint Approach to the Treatment of Chronic Pain, Fatigue, and Stress Disorders
by Mark Seem
ISBN 1-891845-13-6
ISBN 978-1-891845-13-0

AGING & BLOOD STASIS: A New Approach to TCM
Geriatrics by Yan De-xin
ISBN 0-936185-63-6
ISBN 978-0-936185-63-7

A NEW AMERICAN ACUPUNCTURE By Mark Seem
ISBN 0-936185-44-9
ISBN 978-0-936185-44-6

BETTER BREAST HEALTH NATURALLY
with CHINESE MEDICINE
by Honora Lee Wolfe & Bob Flaws
ISBN 0-936185-90-2
ISBN 978-0-936185-90-3

BIOMEDICINE: A Textbook for Practitioners of Acupuncture
and Oriental Medicine
by Bruce H. Robinson, MD
ISBN 1-891845-38-1
ISBN 978-1-891845-38-3

THE BOOK OF JOOK:
Chinese Medicinal Porridges
by B. Flaws
ISBN 0-936185-60-6
ISBN 978-0-936185-60-0

CHANNEL DIVERGENCES
Deeper Pathways of the Web
by Miki Shima and Charles Chase
ISBN 1-891845-15-2
ISBN 978-1-891845-15-4

CHINESE MEDICAL OBSTETRICS
by Bob Flaws
ISBN 1-891845-30-6
ISBN 978-1-891845-30-7

CHINESE MEDICAL PALMISTRY:
Your Health in Your Hand
by Zong Xiao-fan & Gary Liscum
ISBN 0-936185-64-3
ISBN 978-0-936185-64-4

CHINESE MEDICAL PSYCHIATRY
A Textbook and Clinical Manual
by Bob Flaws and James Lake, MD
ISBN 1-845891-17-9
ISBN 978-1-845891-17-8

CHINESE MEDICINAL TEAS: Simple, Proven, Folk Formulas
for Common Diseases & Promoting Health
by Zong Xiao-fan & Gary Liscum
ISBN 0-936185-76-7
ISBN 978-0-936185-76-7

CHINESE MEDICINAL WINES & ELIXIRS
by Bob Flaws
ISBN 0-936185-58-9
ISBN 978-0-936185-58-3

CHINESE MEDICINE & HEALTHY WEIGHT
MANAGEMENT: An Evidence-based Integrated Approach by
Juliette Aiyana, L. Ac.
ISBN 1-891845-44-6
ISBN 978-1-891845-44-4

CHINESE PEDIATRIC MASSAGE THERAPY: A Parent's &
Practitioner's Guide to the Prevention & Treatment of Childhood Illness
by Fan Ya-li
ISBN 0-936185-54-6
ISBN 978-0-936185-54-5

CHINESE SELF-MASSAGE THERAPY:
The Easy Way to Health
by Fan Ya-li
ISBN 0-936185-74-0
ISBN 978-0-936185-74-3

THE CLASSIC OF DIFFICULTIES:
A Translation of the Nan Jing
translation by Bob Flaws
ISBN 1-891845-07-1
ISBN 978-1-891845-07-9

A COMPENDIUM OF CHINESE MEDICAL MENSTRUAL
DISEASES
by Bob Flaws
ISBN 1-891845-31-4
ISBN 978-1-891845-31-4

CONTROLLING DIABETES NATURALLY WITH CHINESE
MEDICINE
by Lynn Kuchinski
ISBN 0-936185-06-3
ISBN 978-0-936185-06-2

CURING ARTHRITIS NATURALLY WITH
CHINESE MEDICINE
by Douglas Frank & Bob Flaws
ISBN 0-936185-87-2
ISBN 978-0-936185-87-3

CURING DEPRESSION NATURALLY WITH
CHINESE MEDICINE
by Rosa Schnyer & Bob Flaws
ISBN 0-936185-94-5
ISBN 978-0-936185-94-1

CURING FIBROMYALGIA NATURALLY WITH
CHINESE MEDICINE
by Bob Flaws
ISBN 1-891845-09-8
ISBN 978-1-891845-09-3

CURING HAY FEVER NATURALLY WITH
CHINESE MEDICINE
by Bob Flaws
ISBN 0-936185-91-0
ISBN 978-0-936185-91-0

CURING HEADACHES NATURALLY WITH
CHINESE MEDICINE
by Bob Flaws
ISBN 0-936185-95-3
ISBN 978-0-936185-95-8

CURING IBS NATURALLY WITH CHINESE
MEDICINE
by Jane Bean Oberski
ISBN 1-891845-11-X
ISBN 978-1-891845-11-6

CURING INSOMNIA NATURALLY WITH
CHINESE MEDICINE
by Bob Flaws
ISBN 0-936185-86-4
ISBN 978-0-936185-86-6

CURING PMS NATURALLY WITH CHINESE
MEDICINE
by Bob Flaws
ISBN 0-936185-85-6
ISBN 978-0-936185-85-9

DISEASES OF THE KIDNEY & BLADDER
by Hoy Ping Yee Chan, et al.
ISBN 1-891845-37-3
ISBN 978-1-891845-35-6

THE DIVINE FARMER'S MATERIA MEDICA
A Translation of the Shen Nong Ben Cao
translation by Yang Shouz-zhong
ISBN 0-936185-96-1
ISBN 978-0-936185-96-5

DUI YAO: THE ART OF COMBINING
CHINESE HERBAL MEDICINALS
by Philippe Sionneau
ISBN 0-936185-81-3
ISBN 978-0-936185-81-1

ENDOMETRIOSIS, INFERTILITY AND
TRADITIONAL CHINESE MEDICINE:
A Laywoman's Guide
by Bob Flaws
ISBN 0-936185-14-7
ISBN 978-0-936185-14-9

THE ESSENCE OF LIU FENG-WU'S
GYNECOLOGY
by Liu Feng-wu, translated by Yang Shou-zhong
ISBN 0-936185-88-0
ISBN 978-0-936185-88-0

EXTRA TREATISES BASED ON INVESTIGATION
& INQUIRY:
A Translation of Zhu Dan-xi's Ge Zhi Yu Lun
translation by Yang Shou-zhong
ISBN 0-936185-53-8
ISBN 978-0-936185-53-8

FIRE IN THE VALLEY: TCM Diagnosis & Treatment of
Vaginal Diseases
by Bob Flaws
ISBN 0-936185-25-2
ISBN 978-0-936185-25-5

FU QING-ZHU'S GYNECOLOGY
trans. by Yang Shou-zhong and Liu Da-wei
ISBN 0-936185-35-X
ISBN 978-0-936185-35-4

FULFILLING THE ESSENCE:
A Handbook of Traditional & Contemporary Treatments for
Female Infertility
by Bob Flaws
ISBN 0-936185-48-1
ISBN 978-0-936185-48-4

GOLDEN NEEDLE WANG LE-TING: A 20th Century
Master's Approach to Acupuncture
by Yu Hui-chan and Han Fu-ru, trans. by Shuai Xue-zhong
ISBN 0-936185-78-3
ISBN 978-0-936185-78-1

A HANDBOOK OF TCM PATTERNS
& THEIR TREATMENTS
by Bob Flaws & Daniel Finney
ISBN 0-936185-70-8
ISBN 978-0-936185-70-5

A HANDBOOK OF TRADITIONAL
CHINESE DERMATOLOGY
by Liang Jian-hui, trans. by Zhang Ting-liang
& Bob Flaws
ISBN 0-936185-46-5
ISBN 978-0-936185-46-0

A HANDBOOK OF TRADITIONAL
CHINESE GYNECOLOGY
by Zhejiang College of TCM, trans. by Zhang Ting-liang
& Bob Flaws
ISBN 0-936185-06-6 (4th edit.)
ISBN 978-0-936185-06-4

A HANDBOOK OF CHINESE HEMATOLOGY
by Simon Becker
ISBN 1-891845-16-0
ISBN 978-1-891845-16-1

A HANDBOOK of TCM PEDIATRICS
by Bob Flaws
ISBN 0-936185-72-4
ISBN 978-0-936185-72-9

THE HEART & ESSENCE OF DAN-XI'S
METHODS OF TREATMENT
by Xu Dan-xi, trans. by Yang Shou-zhong
ISBN 0-926185-50-3
ISBN 978-0-936185-50-7

HERB TOXICITIES & DRUG INTERACTIONS:
A Formula Approach by Fred Jennes with Bob Flaws
ISBN 1-891845-26-8
ISBN 978-1-891845-26-0

IMPERIAL SECRETS OF HEALTH & LONGEVITY
by Bob Flaws
ISBN 0-936185-51-1
ISBN 978-0-936185-51-4

INSIGHTS OF A SENIOR ACUPUNCTURIST
by Miriam Lee
ISBN 0-936185-33-3
ISBN 978-0-936185-33-0

INTEGRATED PHARMACOLOGY: Combining Modern
Pharmacology with Chinese Medicine
by Dr. Greg Sperber with Bob Flaws
ISBN 1-891845-41-1
ISBN 978-0-936185-41-3

INTRODUCTION TO THE USE OF PROCESSED
CHINESE MEDICINALS
by Philippe Sionneau
ISBN 0-936185-62-7
ISBN 978-0-936185-62-0

KEEPING YOUR CHILD HEALTHY WITH
CHINESE MEDICINE
by Bob Flaws
ISBN 0-936185-71-6
ISBN 978-0-936185-71-2

THE LAKESIDE MASTER'S STUDY OF THE PULSE
by Li Shi-zhen, trans. by Bob Flaws
ISBN 1-891845-01-2
ISBN 978-1-891845-01-7

MANAGING MENOPAUSE NATURALLY WITH
CHINESE MEDICINE
by Honora Lee Wolfe
ISBN 0-936185-98-8
ISBN 978-0-936185-98-9

MASTER HUA'S CLASSIC OF THE
CENTRAL VISCERA
by Hua Tuo, trans. by Yang Shou-zhong
ISBN 0-936185-43-0
ISBN 978-0-936185-43-9

THE MEDICAL I CHING: Oracle of the
Healer Within
by Miki Shima
ISBN 0-936185-38-4
ISBN 978-0-936185-38-5

MENOPAIUSE & CHINESE MEDICINE
by Bob Flaws
ISBN 1-891845-40-3
ISBN 978-1-891845-40-6

MOXIBUSTION: The Power of Mugwort Fire
by Lorraine Wilcox
ISBN 1-891845-46-2
ISBN 978-1-891845-46-8

TEST PREP WORKBOOK FOR THE NCCAOM BIO-MEDICINE
MODULE: Exam Preparation & Study Guide
by Zhong Bai-song
ISBN 1-891845-34-9
ISBN 978-1-891845-34-5

POINTS FOR PROFIT: The Essential Guide to Practice Success for Acupuncturists 3rd Edition
by Honora Wolfe, Eric Strand & Marilyn Allen
ISBN 1-891845-25-X
ISBN 978-1-891845-25-3

PRINCIPLES OF CHINESE MEDICAL ANDROLOGY: An Integrated Approach to Male Reproductive and Urological Health
by Bob Damone
ISBN 1-891845-45-4
ISBN 978-1-891845-45-1

PRINCE WEN HUI's COOK: Chinese Dietary Therapy
By Bob Flaws & Honora Wolfe
ISBN 0-912111-05-4
ISBN 978-0-912111-05-6

THE PULSE CLASSIC:
A Translation of the Mai Jing
by Wang Shu-he, trans. by Yang Shou-zhong
ISBN 0-936185-75-9
ISBN 978-0-936185-75-0

THE SECRET OF CHINESE PULSE DIAGNOSIS
by Bob Flaws
ISBN 0-936185-67-8
ISBN 978-0-936185-67-5

SECRET SHAOLIN FORMULAS for the Treatment of
External Injury
by De Chan, trans. by Zhang Ting-liang & Bob Flaws
ISBN 0-936185-08-2
ISBN 978-0-936185-08-8

STATEMENTS OF FACT IN TRADITIONAL
CHINESE MEDICINE   Revised & Expanded
by Bob Flaws
ISBN 0-936185-52-X
ISBN 978-0-936185-52-1

STICKING TO THE POINT: A Step by Step Approach to TCM
Acupuncture Therapy
by Bob Flaws & Honora Lee Wolfe
ISBN 1-891845-47-0
ISBN 978-1-891845-47-5

A STUDY OF DAOIST ACUPUNCTURE &
MOXIBUSTION
by Liu Zheng-cai
ISBN 1-891845-08-X
ISBN 978-1-891845-08-6

THE SUCCESSFUL CHINESE HERBALIST
by Bob Flaws and Honora Lee Wolfe
ISBN 1-891845-29-2
ISBN 978-1-891845-29-1

THE SYSTEMATIC CLASSIC OF ACUPUNCTURE
& MOXIBUSTION
A translation of the Jia Yi Jing
by Huang-fu Mi, trans. by Yang Shou-zhong &
Charles Chace
ISBN 0-936185-29-5
ISBN 978-0-936185-29-3

THE TAO OF HEALTHY EATING ACCORDING TO
CHINESE MEDICINE
by Bob Flaws
ISBN 0-936185-92-9
ISBN 978-0-936185-92-7

TEACH YOURSELF TO READ MODERN
MEDICAL CHINESE
by Bob Flaws
ISBN 0-936185-99-6
ISBN 978-0-936185-99-6

TEST PREP WORKBOOK FOR BASIC TCM THEORY
by Zhong Bai-song
ISBN 1-891845-43-8
ISBN 978-1-891845-43-7

TREATING PEDIATRIC BED-WETTING WITH
ACUPUNCTURE & CHINESE MEDICINE
by Robert Helmer
ISBN 1-891845-33-0
ISBN 978-1-891845-33-8

TREATISE on the SPLEEN & STOMACH: A Translation and
Annotation of Li Dong-yuan's
Pi Wei Lun
by Bob Flaws
ISBN 0-936185-41-4
ISBN 978-0-936185-41-5

THE TREATMENT OF CARDIOVASCULAR
DISEASES WITH CHINESE MEDICINE
by Simon Becker, Bob Flaws &
Robert Casañas, MD
ISBN 1-891845-27-6
ISBN 978-1-891845-27-7

THE TREATMENT OF DIABETES MELLITUS WITH
CHINESE MEDICINE
by Bob Flaws, Lynn Kuchinski &
Robert Casañas, M.D.
ISBN 1-891845-21-7
ISBN 978-1-891845-21-5

THE TREATMENT OF DISEASE IN TCM, Vol. 1: Diseases of
the Head & Face, Including Mental & Emotional Disorders
by Philippe Sionneau & Lü Gang
ISBN 0-936185-69-4
ISBN 978-0-936185-69-9

THE TREATMENT OF DISEASE IN TCM, Vol. II: Diseases of
the Eyes, Ears, Nose, & Throat
by Sionneau & Lü
ISBN 0-936185-73-2
ISBN 978-0-936185-73-6

THE TREATMENT OF DISEASE IN TCM, Vol. III: Diseases
of the Mouth, Lips, Tongue, Teeth & Gums
by Sionneau & Lü
ISBN 0-936185-79-1
ISBN 978-0-936185-79-8

THE TREATMENT OF DISEASE IN TCM, Vol IV: Diseases of
the Neck, Shoulders, Back, & Limbs
by Philippe Sionneau & Lü Gang
ISBN 0-936185-89-9
ISBN 978-0-936185-89-7

THE TREATMENT OF DISEASE IN TCM, Vol V: Diseases of
the Chest & Abdomen
by Philippe Sionneau & Lü Gang
ISBN 1-891845-02-0
ISBN 978-1-891845-02-4

THE TREATMENT OF DISEASE IN TCM, Vol VI: Diseases of
the Urogential System & Proctology
by Philippe Sionneau & Lü Gang
ISBN 1-891845-05-5
ISBN 978-1-891845-05-5

THE TREATMENT OF DISEASE IN TCM, Vol VII: General
Symptoms
by Philippe Sionneau & Lü Gang
ISBN 1-891845-14-4
ISBN 978-1-891845-14-7

THE TREATMENT OF EXTERNAL DISEASES WITH
ACUPUNCTURE & MOXIBUSTION
by Yan Cui-lan and Zhu Yun-long, trans. by Yang Shou-zhong
ISBN 0-936185-80-5
ISBN 978-0-936185-80-4

THE TREATMENT OF MODERN WESTERN
MEDICAL DISEASES WITH CHINESE MEDICINE
by Bob Flaws & Philippe Sionneau
ISBN 1-891845-20-9
ISBN 978-1-891845-20-8

UNDERSTANDING THE DIFFICULT PATIENT: A Guide
for Practitioners of Oriental Medicine
by Nancy Bilello, RN, L.ac.
ISBN 1-891845-32-2
ISBN 978-1-891845-32-1

YI LIN GAI CUO (Correcting the Errors in the Forest
of Medicine)
by Wang Qing-ren
ISBN 1-891845-39-X
ISBN 978-1-891845-39-0

70 ESSENTIAL CHINESE HERBAL FORMULAS
by Bob Flaws
ISBN 0-936185-59-7
ISBN 978-0-936185-59-0

160 ESSENTIAL CHINESE READY-MADE
MEDICINES
by Bob Flaws
ISBN 1-891945-12-8
ISBN 978-1-891945-12-3

630 QUESTIONS & ANSWERS ABOUT CHINESE
HERBAL MEDICINE:
A Workbook & Study Guide
by Bob Flaws
ISBN 1-891845-04-7
ISBN 978-1-891845-04-8

260 ESSENTIAL CHINESE MEDICINALS
by Bob Flaws
ISBN 1-891845-03-9
ISBN 978-1-891845-03-1

750 QUESTIONS & ANSWERS ABOUT ACUPUNCTURE
Exam Preparation & Study Guide
by Fred Jennes
ISBN 1-891845-22-5
ISBN 978-1-891845-22-2